PRAISE FOR THE JOURNEY THROUGH CANCER

"A timely addition to the medical bookshelf....Dr. Geffen lauds the benefits of complementary practices in treating the person as a whole. But he does not advocate swallowing these notions and potions instead of proven treatments. [He tries]...to address the emotional and spiritual needs of his patients and provide traditional care. These efforts will sound refreshing for cancer patients, many of whom feel they are simply cases being run through a treatment mill."

—*New York Times*

"When a 69-year-old friend was recently diagnosed [with cancer]...his family and friends wondered how he would manage his late-stage disease. Dr. Geffen's *The Journey Through Cancer* will be my gift to him to help him on his journey....Dr. Geffen's calm, balanced voice of experience convinced me that he is on to something."

—*Journal of the National Cancer Institute*

"Oncologist Jeremy R. Geffen, M.D., has done medicine—physicians, nurses, allied health providers, patients, and their families—an extraordinary service in giving us this sensitive, thoughtful, beautifully written book."

—*The Integrative Medicine Consult*

"Dr. Jeremy Geffen is an oncologist of the future, one who integrates the best of traditional and nontraditional approaches. He addresses the physical as well as the psychosocial, emotional, and spiritual dimensions of health and healing. It is unfortunate that all people who are concerned with cancer can't have Dr. Geffen as their doctor; this book is the next best thing."

—Dean Ornish, M.D., president of the Preventive Medicine Research Institute and author of *Dr. Dean Ornish's Program for Reversing Heart Disease* and *Love and Survival*

THE

JOURNEY

THROUGH

CANCER

An Oncologist's Seven-Level

Program for Healing and

Transforming the Whole Person

JEREMY R. GEFFEN, M.D.

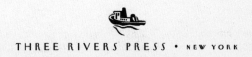

THREE RIVERS PRESS • NEW YORK

Copyright © 2000 by Jeremy Geffen, M.D.

Published by Three Rivers Press, New York, New York.
Member of the Crown Publishing Group.

Random House, Inc. New York, Toronto, London, Sydney, Auckland
www.randomhouse.com

THREE RIVERS PRESS and the Tugboat design are registered trademarks
of Random House, Inc.

Originally published in hardcover by Crown Publishers in 2000.

Printed in the United States of America

Design by Lauren Dong

Library of Congress Cataloging-in-Publication Data
Geffen, Jeremy R., M.D.
    The journey through cancer : an oncologist's seven-level program for healing and
transforming the whole person / Jeremy R. Geffen, M.D.
    Includes bibliographical references.
    1. Cancer—Popular works.   2. Cancer—Alternative treatment.
3. Holistic medicine.   I. Title.
RC263.G426   2000
616.99'406—dc21   99-34017

ISBN 0-609-80704-8

10 9 8 7 6 5 4 3 2 1

First Paperback Edition

DEDICATED TO THE SPIRIT OF FREEDOM

AND LOVE

IN THE HEART OF ALL BEINGS.

AUTHOR'S NOTE

This book is not intended as a substitute for the medical advice of physicians. The reader should regularly consult his or her doctor in matters relating to health, symptoms that may require diagnosis or medical attention, and treatments. Every person is unique, and diagnosis and treatment must be individualized for the reader by his or her doctor.

CONTENTS

IF THE HEALING ART IS MOST DIVINE, IT MUST
OCCUPY ITSELF WITH THE SOUL AS WELL AS WITH
THE BODY.

—APOLLONIUS OF TYANA,
FIRST CENTURY A.D.

THE

JOURNEY
THROUGH
CANCER

INTRODUCTION

WHERE THERE IS NO VISION, THE PEOPLE SHALL
PERISH.

—PROVERBS 29:18

Early in my senior year of medical school, my father was diagnosed with stomach cancer. It was a cool, fall evening—September 18, 1985—and I had just arrived home after a tiring day. Flopping down in a big chair to relax, I casually pressed the PLAY button on my answering machine and was surprised to hear my father's voice. He rarely called.

"Oh, Jeremy," he said with some hesitation, "I think I've got a little problem. I had an endoscopy today and the doctor said I have a tumor in my stomach. Unfortunately, it's malignant. Maybe you could give me a call."

With my heart pounding I picked up the telephone and dialed his number. I knew this was not going to be a little problem. Not at all.

My father's illness occurred at a time when—after many years of distance and great difficulty in our relationship—he and I were falling in love with each other. I was twenty-nine, and like so many men of my generation I had missed a close relationship with my father. He was a tough, distant, romantic dreamer who during my childhood years was so deeply involved in his own struggles that he was unable to function as a parent in any conventional sense. When I was twelve he left our family to pursue his own life and dreams. He eventually built a career in New York City as the owner of two respected repertory cinema theaters and married a French woman who was a film director. They lived a remarkably bohemian life and were well known in the film circles of New York and Europe.

Although I now understand so much more of what occurred during those years, his departure was extremely painful. Still, after many years of challenge and conflict, we had recently, magically, discovered a love for each other that felt as exciting as any love I had ever known. At last, after all these years, I was finally finding my father. And in the process, a deep, old, and hurtful wound was starting to heal.

As it turned out, his newly discovered cancer was an aggressive one. When his stomach was removed the next week we learned that the tumor had already spread into his liver and lymph nodes. "I'm sorry," the surgeon said after the operation, "the tumor was very extensive, and I couldn't get it all. I took out as much as I could. There was nothing more I could do."

Thus from the beginning the situation looked quite bleak. Our entire family felt stunned and completely disoriented, as if we had all been suddenly thrown into a bad dream. I could hardly believe this was happening. And there was a knot in the pit of my stomach that would not go away.

As the gravity of the situation began to sink in, my father's agony and the pain in my own heart and soul penetrated in a way I can hardly describe. After all these years we had finally found each other, and now he was dying. It was too much to accept.

From that time until just before his death three and a half months later, we were partners in trying to find ways to help him fight and live. There was no small irony in the fact that early on in medical school I had decided that I would become an oncologist and dedicate myself to helping individuals and families who were dealing with cancer. Now suddenly, and in a very personal way, I was about to learn more about oncology than I had ever imagined, and much more about the extraordinary journey taken by people with cancer.

As a senior at New York University School of Medicine I had access to the best hospitals and cancer specialists. My father also could afford the best medical care available. As we made the rounds of New York's top cancer centers and oncologists, I became progressively more discouraged by what he was experiencing. He was almost always identified by his tissue diagnosis *(high-grade gastric adenocarcinoma)* and stage of disease *(pathologic Stage IV, with extensive liver and lymph node involvement)*, rather than by who he was as a human being. He was not seen as a *person with cancer*. Rather, from the moment of his diagnosis he was instantaneously and forever more transformed into a *cancer patient*. I had somehow managed to get through three years of medical school without fully understanding how quickly and pervasively this happens, or the effects it can have on those who are sick and on their families. And because of my father's particular diagnosis, he was invariably regarded as someone who was basically already dead. The words METASTATIC GASTRIC CANCER hung like an unpleasant odor in the room each time they were spoken, producing the same unmistakable frown on the face of virtually every oncologist he saw. Chemotherapy was offered, but with little enthusiasm, and always with a similar, unmistakable message—spoken or unspoken—that it probably wouldn't do much good. Instead, it was often gently suggested that it might be best for him to "get his affairs in order."

At no time did anyone even hint that my father himself could influence the outcome of what was happening to him. Nor were any ideas offered as to how he could at least improve the quality of the life he had left to live, regardless of how short a time that might be. Perhaps most distressingly absent of all were any suggestions of what he might do to deal with the mental, emotional, and spiritual aspects of all that he was experiencing: the tremendous fear and sense of loss associated with losing control of his body; the horrible sense of never being able to feel normal again; the loss of his stomach and the radically diminished ability to eat; the loss of his energy and strength; the end of life as he had known it before; and the impending end of his life altogether. Somehow, unbelievably, he was left totally on his own to deal with all of these issues.

All of his family members and friends rallied to his side. However, we were also all dealing with our own pain, sadness, anger, grief, and disbelief. Despite our best efforts, we were unable to find peace of mind in the midst of this traumatic time.

Late one afternoon, after a particularly discouraging visit with his oncologist, my father and I were riding home through Manhattan in a taxi. Some tests had come back that day and the results were not good. Although his oncologist was well intentioned, and I am sure he meant no harm, the clinical, matter-of-fact way in which he had delivered such devastating information was hard to believe. It betrayed precious little awareness—if any—of the impact this was having on my father. And as usual, no meaningful or coherent follow-up support was offered.

During the ride home my father was more quiet and withdrawn than I had ever seen him. As we rode on in silence, I remember how strangely distant and gray the city looked. It was drizzling outside, and the rhythmic sound of the taxi's windshield wipers was all I could hear above the pounding of my heart and the sense of foreboding in my gut. As we began to pass through Central Park, crossing Fifth Avenue at Seventy-second Street, my father suddenly looked at me and began to speak.

"Jeremy," he said, his voice quiet and withdrawn, "I can now see that my doctors have given up on me." He then paused before continuing, almost in a whisper, "How can I have any hope if my doctors have no hope?"

There was a look of resignation and defeat in his eyes that filled me with unimaginable sadness. I remember choking back tears as the deeper meaning of his words sank in.

And in that moment, I saw the light go out of my father's eyes.

Looking back now, I understand that was the moment when my father gave up. Although in the coming weeks he fought on in many ways, I now see how in that moment of despair he decided that his battle had been lost.

How can I have any hope if my doctors have no hope?

His physician's words were now echoing loudly in my own mind, with an unexpected intensity. I was learning—the hard way—how powerful a physician's words could be and the enormous impact they could have on a patient, particularly someone with cancer.

I was also learning, more clearly and more personally than ever before, how the mind, heart, and spirit can profoundly influence the course of a patient's illness, the course of his or her life, and all too often the course of his or her death.

Soon thereafter we began making the rounds of "alternative medicine," embarking on a blind search for *anything* that might help my father have a chance to live. Prior to medical school I had spent six years exploring Eastern religions and philosophy. For four years I lived in an ashram, a spiritual community, where I studied yoga, meditation, and vegetarianism, and learned a great deal about a variety of holistically oriented healing approaches. In addition, between my second and third years of medical school I visited Nepal and India. On that trip, which would be the first of many subsequent journeys to the East, I began to study the ancient and profound medical traditions of India and Tibet—Ayurveda and Tibetan Medicine. I saw the immense power of these traditions to prevent and treat disease and to alleviate the suffering of human beings who are sick. So the next step seemed obvious. If conventional medicine couldn't save my father, maybe Ayurveda could. Or perhaps Tibetan or Chinese herbs. Or perhaps acupuncture, or homeopathic medicine. Or perhaps some special diet. There had to be *something* that would work. And if there was, I was determined to find it. After all, this was my *father*, the one I'd never had before, the one I'd longed for all these years. I couldn't just sit by and let him die.

After seeing a variety of alternative health practitioners, it became increasingly clear that they were well intentioned but remarkably limited in their knowledge of cancer. As a group they also tended to be extremely critical of conventional medicine, as fixed in their own beliefs as they accused the medical profession of being. The herbalists, naturopaths, and Asian medical doctors that my father saw were also emphatic that the chemotherapy he was now taking was "poisoning" him, or "destroying" his immune system. Most refused to treat him as long as he insisted on taking chemotherapy. Sadly, I realized that this was fundamentally no different from the cancer specialists who insisted that they didn't want my father taking any "useless herbs" that might "interfere" with the chemotherapy—even while freely admitting that chemotherapy couldn't cure him anyway.

It was unbelievably frustrating. I felt as if I were stranded in a medical Tower of Babel, surrounded by doctors and healers who were all speaking radically different languages, unwilling and unable to hear or understand one another. Despite our ongoing pleas, they could not or would not look beyond their own particular viewpoints to see if there was anything else that could be done to help my father. Nowhere, it seemed, was there anyone who could provide any meaningful, coherent guidance about where to go, what to do, or how to dig through the avalanche of conflicting information that was coming at us from so many different sources. No one, it seemed, could guide us all the way through the painful and confusing journey we were taking.

Meanwhile, my father was growing weaker. He no longer had any appetite. Every day he lost weight and became steadily more fatigued. Soon it became hard for him to move from his bed. Despite pain pills, shots, herbs, and acupuncture treatments, he was having increased abdominal pain and was vomiting up almost everything he put in his mouth. Nothing was working. We were running out of options, and running out of time. Above all, it was heartbreaking and devastating to see such a vigorous, independent, energetic man deteriorating so quickly.

At this point I began to realize at a deeper level what was really happening. Slowly and reluctantly, I began to face what I had tried with all my heart and mind and soul to avoid: he was going to die, and in fact was already dying. My beloved father was dying, and there was nothing I could do to stop it.

This realization marked the beginning of a major transition in our journey together. For my father, there was a sense of even deeper resignation to the inevitability of his own death. Accepting it was almost a relief for him, because he didn't have to fight anymore. But for me, facing it was extremely difficult because I didn't want to let him go. Deep inside, my heart was crying out, "No! Not now! Not when we have finally found each other after all these years!"

But the reality was inevitable. I had to accept that any further attempts to "help" would only ease my own pain, not his. In fact, urging him to fight on would only add to his burden, not relieve it. He really did not *want* to struggle anymore. He was so exhausted, and life inside his ailing body had simply become too emotionally and physically difficult. Even the simplest things had become overwhelming, and he had finally given up. But I felt so frustrated, even angry. "How can you not want to keep on fighting to live?" my heart demanded. It often took every ounce of self-control not to scream these words out loud.

At this point, trying to hold on to him was like trying to hold water in my hand; like water, he was slipping through my fingers. This was agony.

Intellectually, I knew I couldn't hold on any longer, but emotionally I wasn't ready to let go. No, not yet.

Then one day, in a moment of grace, I saw, and understood, and *accepted* that there was only one thing for me to do. I had to surrender completely to what was happening. No matter how much I wanted to or how hard I tried, I could not change the inevitable outcome. I realized that my greatest challenge now was to love my father as deeply and as fully as possible, while at the same time letting him go. To be there with him fully, but no longer pushing or pulling him in any direction. To let him do completely as he wished in the last days or weeks of his life.

What happened in those last few weeks was profound. It transformed me as a person—and as a physician—in ways that I could not have imagined. As my father's own surrender and acceptance of what was happening deepened, I watched him go through a remarkable transformation—a spiritual awakening that I now recognize as a true healing journey. Though he died soon thereafter, he died with his eyes wide open, embracing the unknown with courage, grace, and love. Most important, our experiences together during the final days and weeks of his life—and in particular one special conversation we had—left no question in my mind that he reached the end of his time on earth with a deep understanding of himself, of life, of death, and of the nature of reality itself.

The incredible intensity of what I had shared with my father propelled me forward in my own journey. I began a deliberate search for greater understanding of all that had happened. I was filled with so many questions, and I felt that I simply had to find the answers—for myself, and for the many patients and families I would see and try to help throughout my life as a doctor.

Just as my experience with my father's illness had been frustrating and painful, I knew other people must be enduring the same thing, or much worse. Few cancer patients have access to the resources that my father did: I was a senior medical student in New York and was knowledgeable about cancer and mainstream medicine. I was also well informed about alternative treatments and had access to many of the best. Furthermore, my father had the desire to explore any treatment option that could conceivably help him. Despite all these advantages, our journey had been excruciatingly difficult and confusing. What must other people go through, I wondered, when they do not have any of these resources to help them? I shuddered thinking of this and felt a deep resolve in my heart to do something about it.

Through my father's experience, I had come to appreciate the profound and universal challenges faced by people with cancer, or any life-threatening disease. In the years since then, this has been repeatedly confirmed by the vast number of cancer patients and family members who have shared their lives, their stories, and their extraordinary journeys with me. So many important concerns had been left unaddressed by my father's physicians during his illness. For instance, there was no meaningful advice about diet and nutrition. Except for recommending more pain and nausea pills, there were no suggestions of things my father could do to help ease his physical discomfort. And there was virtually no discussion of the intense emotional and spiritual issues a human being faces during such a profoundly challenging illness. These are aspects of cancer that the medical profession is only now beginning to address.

I saw too how inadequately my father's problems had been handled by *both* the mainstream and alternative medical systems. It was extremely difficult to find care that was reliable, technically sophisticated, and medically sound—as well as open-minded and knowledgeable about other approaches to healing. Furthermore, it seemed even more difficult to find state-of-the-art medical care offered in an environment that addressed the needs and longings of the mind, heart, and spirit of patients and their families in ways that were meaningful, coherent, and responsible.

From the pain of that experience a conviction began to grow within me that one day I would become the kind of oncologist that I wished so much had been available for my father: someone who understood Western science, but who also understood Eastern medicine and spirituality, as well as other models of healing and consciousness; someone who could look into the mind, heart, and spirit of a human being as intently as he could gaze at an MRI scan or pathology report; someone who provided love, support, wisdom, and hope. A physician who genuinely embraced and lived these philosophies, and who was a truly joyful, spiritually conscious, loving human being. This meant becoming not only a fully credentialed and experienced doctor but a true healer as well. A person dedicated to helping people awaken to their true selves—to the infinite and eternal aspect of their being that is timeless, dimensionless, and untouched by any disease or circumstance.

For more than fourteen years, I have pursued that vision every day. The journey has taken me to many extraordinary places around the world, and through many inner landscapes as well.

Along the way I have been richly blessed. Among the blessings for which I am most grateful is the experience of an intense, extremely high-quality education. I received my undergraduate degree from Columbia University, followed by four years of medical school at New York University School of Medicine. I then had three years of internship and residency training in internal medicine at the University of California at San Diego Medical Center. This was followed by three more years of subspecialty training in hematology and oncology at the University of California at San Francisco Medical Center. These are some of the finest centers of medical education and training in the world. I deeply appreciate and give thanks for the knowledge I gained, the professional training I received, and the many extraordinary people I met.

I have also been blessed over many years by meeting and studying with some of the great spiritual teachers and leading-edge thinkers of our time. Each of them contributed profoundly to my growth and understanding, and their guidance and example has influenced my journey in deep and compelling ways.

The book you're now reading is the result of this journey. The pages that follow present a seven-level program that specifically addresses *all* the aspects of who we are as humans—body, mind, heart, and spirit. In short, *the whole person.* It explores the critically important role that all of these dimensions of ourselves play in the healing process and the extraordinary opportunity we have to understand and embrace them. It also examines the significant role that alternative and complementary approaches to healing and wellness can, and should, play in the care of people with cancer. Finally, it explores the dimension of our true nature that is beyond what can be seen or named. As a physician and as a human being, I believe the vision of this program can truly benefit and inspire us in all areas of life. If you are a cancer patient, family member, or caregiver, you can use this program and draw upon its vision in your own journey, regardless of where you are physically, mentally, emotionally, or spiritually.

Ultimately, the insights I offer here are those I sought for myself—and for the countless patients and family members who have taught me so much, and whose journey through cancer has given so much inspiration and meaning to my own.

1

WHAT IS THE PURPOSE OF MEDICINE?

FOR THIS IS THE GREAT ERROR OF OUR DAY, THAT
PHYSICIANS SEPARATE THE SOUL FROM THE BODY.

—PLATO

In my years of training as a physician and an oncologist, I encountered and absorbed a vast amount of information. I also learned and mastered many different tools, technologies, and clinical skills, and a great many questions were asked and answered. But in all those years of study and preparation, the most fundamental question of all for a physician was never once raised:

What is the purpose of medicine?

Why are we doing this? What exactly are doctors trying to accomplish with all their hard work?

Perhaps it was assumed that everyone knew the answers to these questions: the purpose of medicine is to *fix* people—to replace illness with health. When a patient presents with a problem or symptom of some kind, medicine ought to return the patient to the condition that existed before the problem or symptom occurred. With respect to cancer, the purpose of medicine should be to eradicate tumors, normalize blood tests, alleviate pain, create clear CT scans, and prolong life. These, I believe, are the unspoken, culturally sanctioned notions of what physicians are supposed to do—and as a corollary, these objectives should be accomplished with the least possible effort, expense, and sense of personal responsibility on the part of everyone involved.

Despite its great achievements, the success of modern medicine in achieving these goals remains limited. This is especially true in oncology, where the challenges encountered by patients and family members alike can be extreme. Partly because of these challenges, millions of Americans—and cancer patients in particular—are turning to alternative and complementary forms of medicine. But this trend is not motivated simply by the inability of mainstream doctors to cure their disease. It also arises, I believe, from a fundamental shortsightedness in medicine's understanding of what its purpose should be.

At present, doctors focus primarily on the physical characteristics of their patients—bones and organs, test results, height, weight, and age. Yet in each of us there is a rich mental, emotional, and spiritual reality that influences and even directs the course of our lives. Often, for both patients and their families, cancer brings this inner reality vividly to life and to the surface. If the inner reality is devalued or ignored by modern medicine, the effects can be devastating.

When you are diagnosed with cancer, conventional medicine may respond with surgery, chemotherapy, radiation, or perhaps another leading-edge treatment: in short, whatever is necessary to "get rid of the cancer." Throughout treatment, your physical signs and symptoms are carefully monitored. But many other important areas of your life receive far less attention. How is the illness affecting your marriage, your work, or your ability to find meaning and enjoyment in every day? What are your thoughts, beliefs, fears, and expectations about what will happen to you?

For most doctors and in most hospitals, these questions are of secondary importance. Individual physicians may address these issues, but most feel inadequately trained to handle them competently. As a result, when patients feel anxious or depressed, doctors will often prescribe antianxiety or antidepressant medications. Certainly there are instances in which these medications serve a very important role in the care of people with cancer. But, out of frustration or habit, many physicians rely on them as substitutes for addressing deeper issues.

A doctor's ability to deal with the mental, emotional, and spiritual concerns of his patients is often further restricted by the economics of medicine. Even if physicians have the desire and the skill to spend an hour in meaningful discussion with patients, the health care system in which they are working may make this impossible. In the era of the ten-minute managed care follow-up visit, anything but the most limited cursory assessment is often not possible. The financial, administrative, and time pressures on doctors in America have increased exponentially over the last decade, and current trends in managed health care suggest that things may only get worse.

It's important to mention, too, that a physician who explores emotional issues with patients and families may be opening a Pandora's box of unresolved guilt, anger, hostility, and confusion. Patients' demands and expectations can at times be wildly unrealistic, and disputes with doctors can degenerate into costly, time-consuming, and exhausting litigation. In oncology, where issues of life and death are commonly at stake, and where decisions regarding diagnosis and treatment options can carry huge costs and consequences, emotions often run high. In response, many physicians choose to deal only with technical issues that can be clearly defined, objectified, measured, and treated.

All this often leaves everyone feeling frustrated and dissatisfied. Many doctors simply shut down emotionally and do the best they can under the circumstances. Meanwhile, and in increasing numbers, patients seek out alternative, complementary, and often unproven forms of care.

What is the solution? I believe it's time to enlarge our vision of medicine for cancer patients—and for all patients. In this new vision, medicine has two distinct purposes. The *relative* purpose of medicine is to relieve symptoms and to cure disease. But there is also an *ultimate* purpose, which extends beyond the physical realm to include the mind, heart, and spirit of every patient, and indeed of humanity as a whole.

In this view, cancer patients are understood to be asking two things of their physicians. On the relative level, patients most definitely want their illnesses cured. But this is not the whole story. The ultimate reason *why* they want to be cured is in order to feel love and joy in their lives. Quite often patients are convinced their capacity for this has been violently stripped away by their diagnosis. Many cancer patients believe that they cannot experience the deepest levels of love and joy again until the doctor has gotten rid of the cancer. They have made a decision, consciously or unconsciously, that this physical criterion must be met before they can partake of the profound human emotions we all seek. They feel fundamentally separated from the emotions that make life worth living, and they feel that bridging the separation depends on the clinical work of the doctor.

In light of this, I believe the ultimate purpose of medicine must be to foster the emotional and spiritual fulfillment that is a shared aspiration of all human beings. Moreover, medicine must empower patients to find that fulfillment *within themselves*—regardless of their diagnosis, their current condition, or their clinical outcome.

Thus, I would describe the ultimate purpose of medicine as follows: *to assist all beings to experience unbounded love and joy, and to know this is the essence of who we truly are.* This purpose deserves attention fully equal to the relative purpose of curing disease.

Our potential to experience love and joy is in fact unbounded, and I believe that fulfilling that potential is the true objective of all human activity. But the fullest realization of that objective can never be found in external circumstances—not in a salary, an award, a relationship, or even in a clear CT scan. All external things will eventually change, and sooner or later will disappear. We must recognize, then, that the deepest levels of love, joy, and fulfillment we seek can only be found—and can always be found—*within ourselves.*

Helping patients to discover this is the ultimate purpose of medicine. If this purpose were understood and embraced, so much pain, confusion, and misery could be alleviated, regardless of our success in fulfilling the *relative* purpose of treating disease. Certainly cancer care demands the most advanced technology, and providing that technology for patients is one of my highest priorities. But I also know that no advances in chemotherapy, radiation, surgery—or immunotherapy or gene therapy— can ever fulfill the larger needs and concerns of patients and their families. Even when medicine succeeds in its relative purpose, even when the tumor has been eradicated and the CT scans are clear, our task is not complete unless the ultimate purpose has been fulfilled as well. We must serve every patient's physical needs to the very best of our ability, but we must serve every patient's mind, heart, and spirit as well.

In striving to fulfill both the relative and the ultimate purposes of medicine, I have come to appreciate a fundamental insight that is often overlooked in daily life. In every moment we abide simultaneously in two domains of existence. The domain of *doing* encompasses all our worldly activities, efforts, identities, and endeavors. It includes everything we *do* to try to heal ourselves when we are sick, including taking chemotherapy, radiation, herbs, vitamins, massage, or acupuncture. But there is another domain of existence, the domain of *being,* that is equally real and important. The domain of *being* encompasses *who we really are*—beyond our thoughts, our individual identities, our successes, our failures, our sickness or our health. And the domain of being is where the ultimate purpose of medicine leads.

The chapters that follow present a seven-level program that explores the domains of doing *and* being in our lives. The program is designed to fulfill both the relative and the ultimate purposes of medicine. Most important, it will show you how to embrace *all* the dimensions of who you are as a patient and as a human being, and will promote healing and transformation at the deepest levels of your body, mind, heart, and spirit. Although the program is presented in sequential order, feel free to explore the chapters in any order you wish.

The program begins with a discussion of *The Basics: State-of-the-Art Medical Care,* which I believe must and always will be the foundation of effective cancer treatment.

Level One: Education and Information provides basic information about cancer and current treatment options. This empowers patients to actively participate in and obtain the greatest possible benefit from their care.

Level Two: Psychosocial Support explores the importance of reaching out to others in the journey through cancer.

In *Level Three: The Body as Garden,* patients and family members are invited to see the human body as a growing and evolving whole, a wondrously complex living garden, rather than a machine. This level explores the benefits of good nutrition, exercise, massage, and the full spectrum of other alternative and complementary approaches to healing.

Level Four: Emotional Healing enters the inner realm of the human heart, and the healing power of self-love and forgiveness.

Level Five: The Nature of Mind looks carefully at how our entire experience of life—including life with cancer—is determined by our thoughts, our beliefs, and the meanings we give to events.

Level Six: Life Assessment explores the hopes, goals, and purposes of our lives. What are we living for? What do we want to accomplish, experience, and share with others while we are alive, regardless of how long that might be?

Last, *Level Seven: The Nature of Spirit* embraces the spiritual aspects of the healing process, as well as the dimension of our being that exists beyond illness, beyond even birth and death.

As a physician, this is the vision of medicine and healing that I seek to bring to my patients. My intention is that through this book you will be able to participate in this vision, here and now, regardless of where you live and no matter where you may be on the journey through cancer. I am confident that the time is coming when all patients, and all of medicine, will settle for nothing less.

2

BEVERLY IS EVERY ONE OF US

EVERY TRUTH PASSES THROUGH THREE STAGES
BEFORE IT IS RECOGNIZED. IN THE FIRST, IT IS
RIDICULED. IN THE SECOND, IT IS OPPOSED. IN
THE THIRD, IT IS REGARDED AS SELF-EVIDENT.
—ARTHUR SCHOPENHAUER

"Dr. Geffen, you have a long-distance call on line six."

Debbie Dickerson, CLNI, the new-patient coordinator at our cancer center, was paging me over the intercom. Since it was the middle of a very busy afternoon, I knew it must be important.

Hurrying back to my office, I picked up the phone and heard a frightened female voice.

"Hello, Dr. Geffen. Thank you for taking my call. I'm so sorry to bother you like this, but I just had to talk to you. My name is Beverly Martin. I'm forty-four years old, and I'm calling from New Jersey. *I've just been diagnosed with breast cancer, and I'm terrified.* I had a lump in my breast, and it turned out to be malignant. Last week I had a mastectomy, and it's spread into my lymph nodes. My doctor told me it is a high-grade infiltrating ductal carcinoma, and thirteen of nineteen axillary lymph nodes are positive. He says I'm going to need chemotherapy and radiation, but I'm so frightened. I've heard such awful things about chemotherapy and radiation, and I don't know what to do. I've never been sick a day in my life. I don't understand why this is happening, or where to turn. My friend Phyllis heard you speak at a conference in Los Angeles last fall, and she told me I just had to call you. She said you'd know what to do. Will you help me? Is there any way I can deal with this other than chemotherapy and radiation? I'm so frightened and confused."

Listening intently, I took a deep breath. This woman was a complete stranger, but I recognized her fear and pain all too well. I'd seen and heard it in hundreds of newly diagnosed cancer patients, all of whom had suddenly been presented with the greatest challenge of their lives.

Calls like this come in almost every day. Indeed, they seem to be increasing in number, for reasons that are clear.

Cancer is a growing presence in our society. If heart disease was the affliction of the World War II generation, cancer is becoming the disease of the baby boomers—and more and more people like Beverly, ready or not, are suddenly being forced to confront it.

CANCER STATISTICS IN THE UNITED STATES

It is now estimated that nearly half of all American men and more than a third of all American women who are alive today will be diagnosed with cancer at some point in their life. Each year more than 1.2 million Americans learn they have cancer—more than 3,200 people every single day. And every day over 1,500 people die from the disease.

Cancer is now the second leading cause of death in the United States, behind heart disease. Reports project, however, that cancer may soon surpass heart disease as the leading cause of death in America. In 1999, over 563,000 Americans died from it.

A number of factors have contributed to the increasing mortality from cancer in our country, including a growing population, reduced deaths from heart disease, and the fact that more people are living longer than ever before. Another reason for the rising number of cancer deaths is the increased incidence of certain cancers over the last half of the twentieth century, notably lung and colorectal cancer. There were also significant increases in non-Hodgkin's lymphomas, bladder cancer, liver cancer, and melanomas of the skin.

The increase in prostate cancer—which in 1994 surpassed breast cancer as the most commonly diagnosed malignancy in the United States, after skin cancer—has been even more dramatic. In 1985, there were 85,000 cases of prostate cancer diagnosed in this country. By 1995, the number had climbed to over 244,000 cases, and over 40,000 men died from the disease. A significant percentage of that increase has been attributed to improvements in prostate cancer screening, and since 1995 the number of men diagnosed each year has declined. However, a man in the United States is still estimated to have a 1-in-5 chance of being diagnosed with prostate cancer in his lifetime.

Awareness of the alarming incidence of breast cancer has also grown steadily in the United States in recent years. In 1999 over 176,000 women were diagnosed with breast cancer, and nearly 44,000 women died from the disease. Most American women are now well aware that they have a 1-in-8 chance of developing breast cancer by age eighty-five.

THE ECONOMIC IMPACT OF CANCER IN THE UNITED STATES

In 1985, the National Center for Health Statistics estimated the total cost of cancer in this country at $72.5 billion. By 1990, this cost approached $100 billion, and over the last decade it has continued to rise. Cancer now consumes over 10 percent of the entire health care budget in the United States.

The rising economic impact of cancer is attributable not only to the growing number of cases. Many people are living much longer with the disease and require evaluation and monitoring with expensive technologies such as CT scans, MRI scans, PET scans, and sophisticated blood tests. As treatments become more sophisticated, they often become more expensive as well. For example, in recent years high-dose chemotherapy with peripheral stem cell transplantation has been used for an increasing number of solid tumors as well as hematologic malignancies—and it generally costs tens of thousands of dollars per patient. There has also been tremendous growth in the use of expensive drugs such as G-CSF (Neupogen) and erythropoietin (Procrit, or EPO). These are natural hormones, also known as *growth factors*, that stimulate the production of red and white blood cells. Originally, these drugs were available only in universities and at major medical centers and were used sparingly. But they soon proved so beneficial that they are now routinely used in oncologists' offices all across America.

Over the past several years there has been an unprecedented increase in new cancer drugs approved and released by the FDA for the care and treatment of cancer patients. Hundreds of new drugs are currently in the clinical research pipeline, and these will be steadily released in the future. Almost without exception, they are powerful technologies that have been and will continue to be immensely helpful to many patients. But they will also add to the overall expense of cancer care in our country.

All this illustrates an important point. If a new vision of medicine that honors and cares for the mind, heart, *and* spirit of human beings, as well as their bodies, could even slightly improve the incidence, morbidity, or mortality from cancer—or at the very least reduce the costs of cancer care, or the *suffering* experienced by cancer patients and families—this would translate into tremendous benefits for millions of people in our country and across the world.

The growing interest in alternative and complementary medicine suggests that such a new vision is already coming into being. A landmark 1993 article in the *New England Journal of Medicine* pointed out that in 1990 approximately one-third (33.8 percent) of all Americans used some kind of alternative or complementary therapy in their daily lives. A follow-up to this article, published in the *Journal of the American Medical Association* in November 1998, revealed that in 1997 the utilization of alternative and complementary forms of medicine had risen even further, to 42.1 percent of all Americans. Extrapolations to the U.S. population also suggested a 47.3 percent increase in total visits to alternative and complementary practitioners over a seven-year period of time—from 427 million in 1990 to 629 million in 1997—which exceeded the total visits to all U.S. primary care physicians.

While this trend touches all areas of health care, it is particularly prevalent among cancer patients. The subject of "unconventional cancer therapies" has been covered extensively in the media. From all the statistics and anecdotes, I believe two points are especially important.

First, numerous studies have shown that up to 50 percent of all cancer patients utilize at least one form of unconventional therapy at some point in their illness, and this number will undoubtedly increase in the coming years.

The second point is very disturbing: *Most patients do not disclose their use of alternative or complementary therapies to their medical oncologist.* They are doing these treatments in secret. When trust between patients and physicians is eroded, this in itself can be a serious impediment to the healing process. In addition, lack of open and honest communication can be medically dangerous for patients who may not understand that adverse interactions can occur between various kinds of therapies.

Why is this happening? Why are so many people exploring alternative and complementary approaches to cancer, often at great expense to themselves? Moreover, why are they so often not discussing it with their physicians?

Despite the tremendous advances in cancer detection and treatment in recent years, conventional medicine is still unable to cure many patients with cancer. When confronted with what may be considered by conventional medicine to be an "incurable disease," patients and family members will often turn to alternative or complementary methods in their search for hope.

Many patients are frightened by the rigors and challenges they may encounter as part of conventional cancer treatment, so they seek out forms of care that might be less arduous, less invasive, and less toxic— even if those alternatives might be less effective as well.

Also, many patients and family members turn to alternative or complementary methods because they are seeking a system of care that is more sensitive to their needs *as a whole person.* They want care and attention for their mind, heart, and spirit *as well as* their body.

A new kind of cancer patient is indeed beginning to appear. These are people whose expectations of medicine are very high—not only in terms of clinical treatment but also in their demand that physicians communicate clearly, honestly, and compassionately. When patients seek out alternative and complementary therapies, it is often because they believe they will be listened to, cared for, and *heard.* If there is one lesson that conventional medicine can learn from alternative and complementary therapies, it is the importance of listening attentively to patients and enlisting their participation at every level of the healing process.

The nature of the discussion between a cancer patient and his or her doctor has undergone considerable evolution in the last several decades. In the past the general consensus was that people were better off not knowing the whole truth about their condition. Even direct questions were often deflected with ambiguous responses from doctors and nurses. For a variety of reasons, the situation is now completely different.

One of the most important reasons for this change is a dramatic evolution in cultural beliefs, which now emphasize a patient's "right to know." The notion of "informed consent," which must be unambiguously fulfilled before any medical procedures are performed, is now the cultural as well as the legal standard.

Another obvious reason for the changes in the nature of discussions between patients and doctors is the availability of so many more options. These include sophisticated innovative surgical procedures, advanced radiation therapy techniques, and complex chemotherapy therapy regimens. However, these carry new risks and potential side effects, which must be explained and discussed. Finally, amid all these choices, and despite the clear advances in many areas of cancer treatment, the best option for a particular patient is often not clear. Along with the stress and fear of a cancer diagnosis, the resulting uncertainty can be extremely difficult for patients and family members alike.

Beverly, whom we met at the beginning of this chapter, found herself confronting this kind of situation following her surgery. There were a number of paths she could follow, ranging from no further treatment to pursuing alternative and complementary medicine therapies, from conventional chemotherapy and radiation all the way up to the option of high-dose chemotherapy with stem cell transplantation. She could also try to somehow integrate all these options. Although many people offered Beverly advice, no one could provide her with absolutely clear assurances one way or another. Ultimately she would have to consider her options, review the statistics and reports that were available, consider

the advice and opinions of her doctors, family, and friends, and then…
she had to make her own choice.

A week after our initial telephone conversation, Beverly came to see
me for a consultation. She desperately wanted advice and counsel from a
physician who was not only experienced and knowledgeable about conventional cancer treatments but would also be willing to help her explore
other options. She felt frustrated because she hadn't been able to find
anyone who would guide her through *all* the options. And she was certain of one thing: the stakes of making a "wrong" decision were high.

After we talked for a while, Beverly asked me a very direct question.
"What would you do, Dr. Geffen, if this were you, or your sister, or your
wife?"

Her question was a powerful one, but not unexpected. Whenever I
counsel a cancer patient, this is a touchstone that I always use: *What
would I do if this were me, or a member of my own family?* Fortunately, in
Beverly's case, I felt clear about what I would do, so it was relatively easy
for me to respond.

I could see that she was somewhat surprised by my answer. She knew
by now of my strong belief that cancer treatment should include mental,
emotional, and spiritual components—with a variety of appropriate
complementary therapies for the body as well. She may have expected
that I would suggest forgoing the conventional medical treatments. But,
while acknowledging the limitations of chemotherapy and radiation
therapy, I explained my strong belief that these modalities, when used
skillfully and sensibly—and with love, compassion, wisdom, and
humility—can be extraordinarily beneficial.

"I would do everything," I said. "I would do chemotherapy and radiation, and I would also investigate the latest research on stem cell transplantation in breast cancer. There are also many other things I would do
in terms of diet, nutrition, and exercise. And I would do *everything possible* to explore the deeper dimensions of who I am as a human being, and
the deeper dimensions of healing the body, mind, heart, and spirit.

"You see, Beverly," I continued, "it is true that you have a physical
body, and your body needs love, care, and attention. There is no question
that this is very important, and that it can and will get handled. But you

are a *whole person,* and you have a mind, a heart, and a spirit that need love, care, and attention as well. I believe that honoring and caring for these other aspects of yourself is *just as important* as caring for your body.

"Whatever you do," I concluded, "in the midst of your treatment—including chemotherapy and radiation—or whatever alternative or complementary therapies you might also use, don't forget to find out what is most important to you in life. And above all, don't forget to find out *who you really are.*"

Fortunately, Beverly had a bit of time before making her decision, which is true for most, but not all, patients. She and her family had decided to take a brief vacation to think things over together. I thought this was a great idea, and I encouraged her to spend some of her time sitting quietly and listening to her heart. I suggested that she start writing her thoughts and feelings in a journal every day, including any questions that might come up, and I asked her to call me if she wanted to discuss anything further. At the end our of meeting she thanked me and promised to be in touch again soon.

Beverly embodies and expresses all the strengths and vulnerabilities of the contemporary cancer patient. In a later chapter, we'll meet her again and see how her fear and sense of isolation were transformed into a very different experience—mentally, emotionally, and spiritually. It is important that we learn from Beverly in this way, because as the statistics clearly show, cancer is an extremely widespread disease. Once we understand this, we'll see that Beverly is much more than a typical cancer patient. Beverly is every one of us.

3

THE BASICS:
STATE-OF-THE-ART
MEDICAL CARE

EXCELLENCE, THEN, IS NOT AN ACT, BUT A HABIT.
—ARISTOTLE

This brief chapter exists to make a very important point. It is my absolute conviction that every cancer patient should receive state-of-the-art medical care, administered by an impeccably trained and thoroughly qualified team of caregivers, under the meticulous supervision of an experienced oncologist. This must be the foundation of every cancer treatment program.

Within that general conviction are several additional points that must be made. It is important to address the suspicion and hostility with which many cancer patients, particularly younger ones, approach conventional cancer treatment. A mythology of war stories has grown up around the triad of surgery, chemotherapy, and radiation therapy, which are often called poisonous or even barbaric. There is no doubt that many people have indeed experienced a great deal of pain, frustration, and toxicity associated with these therapies. And this has led some patients to avoid or abandon conventional medicine altogether. However, I believe it is almost always a serious mistake for patients to rely solely on unproven alternative therapies as their primary cancer treatment.

First, there are many instances in the course of care for cancer patients when a decisive medical intervention—especially when performed early in the diagnosis—can literally mean the difference between life and death. Missing such an opportunity because of fears or mistaken ideas about conventional treatment is tragic.

Second, for all the drawbacks and limitations of conventional medicine, alternative or complementary modalities of care can offer nothing that even remotely matches the proven benefits of conventional medicine in treating cancer—particularly on a consistent, reliable basis. Even the great medical traditions of the East, including Ayurveda, Chinese medicine, and Tibetan medicine, clearly acknowledge their own limitations once a disease process has become well established, as it usually has by the time cancer symptoms are manifest.

This is not to suggest that alternative and complementary therapies do not have significant benefits to offer patients, which they most certainly do. But there is an important distinction between therapies intended to treat the *illness* directly and those intended to help treat the *person* who has the illness. At present there are few, if any, scientifically proven benefits of alternative or complementary therapies as a direct treatment for cancer, despite anecdotal evidence to the contrary. Thus, while it is possible that some patients may indeed benefit from alternative and complementary cancer therapies, to choose them exclusively over proven conventional treatment remains a risky proposition.

There is really no reason why conventional medical care and other approaches to healing should be considered mutually exclusive. In fact, it is becoming increasingly recognized that great benefits can be achieved when they are integrated in a thoughtful, rational way. I believe the proper role of these other approaches is as *adjuncts* to conventional care. It is absolutely clear that the treatment options now offered by conventional medicine are safer, less toxic, and far more effective than ever before—and are getting better all the time.

For example:

• A number of cancers that were routinely considered deadly less than 25 years ago, including Hodgkin's disease, testicular cancer, hairy cell leukemia, and childhood leukemia, are curable in the majority of cases, and up to half of all patients with non-Hodgkin's lymphoma can now be cured.

• Postoperative treatment has resulted in a 25 to 30 percent reduction in deaths from locally advanced breast or colorectal cancer.

• Advances in the chemotherapy treatment of multiple myeloma over just the past decade alone have led to a significant improvement in overall survival in patients with this disease.

• Treatment of chronic myelogenous leukemia with newer agents, including alpha-interferon, has also led to dramatic improvements in overall survival compared with just ten years ago.

• At one time a diagnosis of acute myeloid leukemia (AML) was virtually a death sentence. But now more than half of all AML patients treated with chemotherapy achieve a complete remission.

• The preservation of anatomy and function has been greatly advanced in the treatment of many cancers, including those of the eye, breast, larynx, esophagus, rectum, anus, and prostate.

• The addition of chemotherapy to surgery has significantly enhanced survival in the treatment of osteogenic sarcoma (a form of bone cancer), and chemotherapy plus radiation or surgery can now cure a majority of patients with Ewing's sarcoma (another form of bone cancer).

• Recent advances in the treatment of non-small-cell lung cancer with the combination of newer chemotherapy drugs, radiation, and advanced surgical techniques are now extending life in many patients beyond what was considered possible just a few years ago.

• Significant advances have also been made in the area of pain control. New medications, implantable pumps, and more sophisticated surgical interventions give many patients more freedom from pain than ever before.

There is abundant reason to believe that progress against cancer will be even more dramatic in the near future. Entirely new classes of treatment are emerging, many of which are grounded in stunning breakthroughs in molecular and genetic technology. Over the past twenty years, important new understanding of cancer development has been gained through research on:

• *Oncogenes,* which promote the growth of cancer cells
• *Tumor-suppressor genes,* which must function effectively if cancer growth is to be forestalled

- *DNA damage and repair,* which plays a central role in the formation and longevity of cancer cells
- *Angiogenesis,* the ability of tumors to generate the blood vessels which are necessary to provide themselves with vital nutrients
- *Metastasis,* the process by which tumors spread throughout the body
- *Apoptosis,* the mechanisms that regulate the programmed life span of cells.

Advances in these areas are now enabling physicians to attack the disease process at its most fundamental levels. Furthermore, the Human Genome Project, which involves the mapping of the three billion units of encoded genetic information contained in every human cell, is expected to be completed in the first years of the new century. When this is accomplished doctors will be able to create even more powerful treatments that are closely matched to a patient's individual genetic makeup.

For the present, surgery, chemotherapy, and radiation—while admittedly imperfect—are still the most effective treatments for cancer available. Great gains have also been made in recent years in controlling the side effects of chemotherapy. When chemotherapy is carefully administered and monitored, nausea and vomiting now only rarely occur. Sophisticated techniques—including the use of growth factors and stem cell transplantation—allow oncologists to safely administer higher doses of chemotherapy. This significantly lowers the chances of relapse in many patients and provides cures for many others.

Today there are roughly eight million living Americans who at one time have been diagnosed with cancer. Roughly five million of those people have been alive for more than five years since their diagnosis, and the majority of those five million are considered cured. Virtually all of them owe their lives to the achievements of conventional medicine.

New developments in gene therapy, immunotherapy, and other emerging fields may soon race far ahead of current treatments. Gene therapy is an area in which extremely exciting developments are taking place, especially with the discovery of increasing numbers of oncogenes and tumor suppressor genes over the last decade. Likely hundreds of these genes are in every human cell, and the location and function of dozens have already been identified. Mutations of one important tumor-suppressor gene, called *p53*, have been linked to up to 70 percent of colon cancers and are very prevalent in a wide variety of other human cancers. Another well-known oncogene, *HER-2/neu*, has been found to be overexpressed in approximately 30 percent of breast cancers. Understanding of this oncogene has already led to significant changes in the way some patients are being treated for breast cancer.

As our knowledge of these all-important genes and other biochemical processes advances, a true understanding of the molecular basis of cancer will become clear for the first time. Soon it may even be possible to insert a healthy gene into a cell to replace or compensate for damaged genetic material. When this is achieved we will be dealing with the causes of cancer at a deeper level than we ever have before. This will not be just pouring water on the fire of a growing cancer. It will be removing the fuel that the fire needs in order to burn.

Immunotherapy, which uses the body's own defense mechanisms against cancer, holds the promise of creating vaccines against malignancies similar to those for measles, polio, and other formerly widespread diseases. The ability of malignant cells to bypass the body's immune defenses is a key reason why cancer is such a dangerous illness, but for the first time there seems to be real hope that this mystery will be solved. Effective immunotherapies require an ability to identify specific markers, called *antigens*, which differentiate between malignant and normal cells. Once these antigens are identified, they can become targets for immune activity. With new and more effective techniques for identifying tumor antigens, there is real optimism that immunotherapy may soon live up to its promise. In addition, another entirely new class of medications for cancer is emerging that is also directed against tumor antigens. These are called "monoclonal antibodies," of which two examples are already commercially available: Herceptin for breast cancer, and Rituxan for non-Hodgkin's lymphoma.

In addition to these advances, vastly more sophisticated techniques are now being used in the search for other entirely new anticancer drugs. Extremely powerful computers, along with new insights into the inner workings of cells, are enabling researchers to design specific drugs from scratch, rather than having to search for them in nature or among laboratory chemicals. This process, called "rational drug design," is an extraordinary advance in the history of medicine. It holds great promise for the treatment of cancer and virtually all other diseases.

What is leading-edge research today will be routine cancer treatment tomorrow. The emerging modalities are so powerful and fundamental they are certain to shift the very foundations of medicine. As this process takes place, patients' basic perceptions and responses to cancer will also transform. There is no question in my mind that we are now at the threshold of this transformation—and, indeed, have already begun to step through the door.

4

LEVEL ONE:
EDUCATION AND INFORMATION

NOTHING IN LIFE IS TO BE FEARED. IT IS ONLY TO
BE UNDERSTOOD.

—MARIE CURIE

When you are diagnosed with cancer, questions instantly begin to flood your mind. At times, these can be overwhelming....

What is this illness? How did I get it? What will happen to me? Where should I go for treatment? How am I going to pay for it? Does my doctor really know what's going on? Does he or she really care about me? Will I be in pain? Will I be disfigured? Am I going to lose my hair? Will my family and friends still care about me? Am I going to die?

On the journey through cancer, it is vitally important for these and many other questions to be answered accurately, sensitively, and appropriately for your individual needs. Intense fears and beliefs about cancer, even if they are not entirely accurate, can profoundly influence every aspect of the experience. The process is further complicated by the vast amount of information about cancer and cancer therapies that is now available.

In the midst of all this, there is a certain amount of basic information that can be of immense benefit to patients and their family members. Level One of this program is intended to provide that information in a succinct and coherent way.

If your mind is filled with doubts and worries about basic aspects of your medical care, it will be impossible for you to make the best choices about your treatment or derive maximum benefit from it. At the very least, it is important for you to feel confident about the medical care you are receiving. Without this, you will be plagued by fears and anxieties that can adversely affect your healing. You may also risk side effects, treatment delays, or other complications that can be avoided by a basic understanding of your care.

Once these fundamental questions are answered you can begin to explore the deeper dimensions of healing.

The disease we call cancer actually includes more than one hundred different illnesses, each with a different presentation, natural history, and treatment approach. Patients affected by one of the many different forms of cancer are themselves very different from one another. The point at which a diagnosis is made also varies from patient to patient.

Two patients, for example, may receive identical diagnoses, but the fact that their illnesses have the same name is often much less significant than the particular biological features of their tumor and the extent to which the tumor has progressed. Differences in their overall physical condition, their emotional makeup, their support network, and their beliefs and expectations about cancer treatment are also important. These two patients may have entirely different experiences during their illness, and their outcomes may differ as well.

Although cancer is usually described as a war and is often discussed—by doctors, institutions, the public, and the media—using military terminology, I often encourage people to think of cancer as a journey—say, a rafting trip down a river. Sometimes the river can be relatively easy and slow; at other times there are sharp turns and frightening rapids. Like all journeys, different travelers begin at different points on the river, with different levels of knowledge and experience.

In order to get to your destination it is essential to know what sort of river you are traveling on, and where on the river you are starting. You will also need an experienced guide who has navigated this river many times before: someone who knows its twists and turns, and how to best support you along the way. This guide, of course, is your oncologist, and the relationship between you and your doctor is extremely important. But the journey down the river also requires the participation of your companions and the crew of your raft. Your companions are your family members, friends, and associates. The crew includes the medical support staff who are involved in your care, including nurses, phlebotomists, laboratory and radiation technicians, receptionists, billing and insurance staff, and social workers.

As with your doctor, you should be very aware of the profound effect your companions and crew members can have on your journey. If the people beside you in the boat are angry or rushed, if they're impatient or distracted, or if they're not really loving their work, it will influence the quality of your experience in a significant way.

Be especially alert to the beliefs and feelings of your caregivers. Do they share the philosophy that cancer treatment is a journey, or, at the very least, an opportunity for learning and spiritual growth? Or do they see it as an ordeal, or a punishment to be endured? Although it may be challenging for a new patient to understand, the journey through cancer should not be rushed. It is important to take an appropriate amount of time to make informed, empowered decisions. It is also helpful to stop at various places along the way to look over the terrain, to reflect on what's really happening, and to see what you can learn from the entire experience.

I hope it's becoming clear that the experience of cancer includes much more than the technical aspects of medical care. Your relationships with family, friends, and caregivers will play a vital role. Careful choice of your doctor and awareness of the environment in which you are treated are also vitally important. Your medical team should certainly be technically competent, but they must also clearly demonstrate that they truly care about you as a unique human being.

"I'VE JUST BEEN DIAGNOSED WITH CANCER. WHAT SHOULD I DO?"

Upon receiving a cancer diagnosis, you may find yourself facing this frightening experience without any knowledge or understanding of how best to help yourself. The sheer volume of information that is now available about cancer and various treatment options can make the aftermath of diagnosis even more distressing for you and your family. The appropriate answers to your questions are unique to you and your specific circumstances, and they should come directly from your physician. However, a few basic principles can help everyone who faces this challenge:

1. Recognize that fear is natural, and know that it can be overcome.

For the great majority of patients, there is a sharp and very understandable focus on the physical aspects of the illness and treatment process. An important message of this book bears repeating here: *The mental, emotional, and spiritual aspects of cancer are often as immediate, urgent, and challenging—if not more so—than the physical concerns.* By understanding and recognizing fear as a completely normal reaction, you can begin to develop the conviction that it can and will be overcome. Recognize your need for love, support, and highly reliable information and know that you can and will find it. No matter how scared or confused you may be feeling, you must consciously choose to believe that you will get the care and support that you need and deserve. Decide right now to seek out and utilize the many sources of comfort and emotional support that can so greatly benefit you at this time. You will be amazed by the number of loving, caring individuals, organizations, and groups that are ready and willing to help. Information about these is provided in the appendices at the end of this book. But you must be open and willing to receive what they have to offer. Once again: decide right now to give yourself the gift of love and support that can be so precious at this critical time.

2. Slow down the decision-making process.

In the initial phase of dealing with cancer, you may feel a sense of urgency to decide what kind of surgery, chemotherapy, radiation therapy, or other treatments you should have. You may also want to know about taking herbs, vitamins, and supplements, and about how you should change your diet—and you will want this information *immediately*. Very few instances exist in cancer treatment, however, in which such urgency is warranted. The process can almost always be slowed down for at least a few days in order to gather information and support. Don't allow yourself to be frightened or pressured into making any decisions about your treatment until you have a clear understanding of your choices. Take time to explore your options. Take time to breathe—and breathe deeply!

3. Ask yourself this question: Do I have trust and confidence in my doctor?

In order to safely and effectively navigate your way through the diagnosis and treatment of cancer, you must have a qualified guide. In my opinion, this guide should be a well-trained oncologist who is experienced in dealing with your particular kind of cancer. In addition, you should feel assured that your doctor cares about you as an individual, and that he or she truly has your best interests at heart. Your doctor must also be able to readily take care of you if you become sick. What kind of hospital or medical center is the doctor affiliated with? What other specialists are available, if needed? Where will you go if you have problems or complications from your illness or treatment? Is this an environment in which you feel safe, comfortable, and genuinely cared for?

In many instances, dealing with cancer is straightforward, and the course to follow is clear. Sometimes, however, the best course is not clear at all—a wide array of options and treatment approaches exist for many cancers. Each has its own advantages, disadvantages, risks, benefits, and potential toxicities, and appreciating these distinctions will take time and careful consideration. In such cases, it is important to communicate openly and directly with your doctor, and to have all your questions and concerns adequately addressed. If you feel this is not happening, you should by no means compromise. You must find and choose a doctor you can talk to, who genuinely respects your viewpoint, feelings, and wishes. This may require interviewing a number of oncologists. Don't hesitate to get a second opinion, or as many opinions as you need, until you feel at ease with your doctor and the options presented to you. Your relationship with your oncologist may become one of the most important relationships in your life, so make sure you are comfortable and confident before you proceed.

4. Recognize that your physical body needs love and attention, but so do your mind, heart, and spirit.

Cancer is most certainly a crisis that is occurring in the physical body, and it is imperative that patients receive the best possible medical care for their disease. Once again, this care must be guided by a competent, caring, and qualified guide, and administered in an impeccable manner. Integrating other modalities such as nutrition, exercise, vitamins, herbs, supplements, acupuncture, and massage can also be extremely important and valuable. But while you *have* a body, who you are is not limited to your body. You are *a whole person*. Thus, for healing to be complete, *all* the dimensions of who you are as a human being must be addressed with *equal* skill and attention—including your mind, heart, and spirit. Take time every single day to honor and care for these other dimensions of who you are.

5. Recognize that life is a journey, and so is dealing with cancer.

All of life has a rhythm, a natural unfolding, and this includes the experience of cancer. It is important to seek out the information and care that you need. But it is equally important to remember that you need time to rest, to relax, to experience silence, and to be still. Give yourself this time each and every day. It is also important to give yourself permission to feel what you feel. Don't judge yourself—in any way—for whatever you may be experiencing at this moment in time. Know that dealing with cancer is a process in which you can and will become skilled and masterful. Recognize the fact that right now more resources exist to help and guide you than ever before in history, and these resources are fully available to you. You can find what you need, and you will.

FOUR MAJOR CATEGORIES OF CANCER PATIENTS

Four categories of patients journey through cancer, and all of these patients have similar hopes, fears, needs, and concerns. Understanding which of the four major groups you belong to can help you and your family members resist the panic reflex that is so often activated by the word *cancer*.

1. Newly diagnosed patients who have not yet had surgery or begun other treatments

New diagnostic techniques, screening methods, and heightened awareness of cancer risks are changing not only the needs and concerns of cancer patients but also their clinical profiles. In an increasing number of new patients, cancer is far less advanced and far less life-threatening than in the past. Cancer of the prostate, breast, lung, and colon are, in descending order, the most commonly diagnosed forms of the disease. In early stages, each of these, and many other forms of cancer, are potentially curable by surgery alone.

Currently about 50 percent of all people who are diagnosed with cancer will be cured with surgery. More than half of all colon cancer patients, for example, will have their early-stage tumors removed and the disease will not reappear. Other kinds of cancer may also become surgically curable following initial treatment with chemotherapy or radiation (called *neo-adjuvant* therapy).

This extremely positive news is tempered by two other realities. First, 600,000 people per year in the United States are not cured with surgery. Second, all too often surgically treated patients live in fear that the disease will return. Although their cancer is gone, they may be no better informed about how diet, exercise, and other factors can affect their health.

2. Patients who have undergone surgery and are being advised to have further treatment

Following cancer surgery, many cancer patients are advised to receive additional treatment with chemotherapy, radiation, or both (called *adjuvant* therapy) to prevent or diminish the chances of recurrence. For example, a woman who has undergone a lumpectomy for breast cancer is usually advised to have radiation to the remaining breast tissue. She may also be told that she needs four to six months of chemotherapy, and very likely five years of tamoxifen as well. Following surgery for colon cancer, a patient may be advised that he needs chemotherapy lasting up to six months. Similar therapies are now commonly recommended for patients who have undergone surgery for cancers of the head and neck, lung, ovaries, uterus, and bladder, among others.

Many patients regard these treatments with almost as much fear and anger as they have for the disease itself. Again, these feelings often appear reflexively, from associations with horror stories they have heard over the years. Perhaps a breast cancer patient has read an article describing chemotherapy as poisoning the body with chemicals to cleanse it of disease. Or a man with colon cancer may read that chemotherapy is like dropping a bomb on a battlefield in the hope it will kill more bad guys than good guys.

I would like to make three important points concerning these fears:

First, fear is a poor starting point for decision making. It can cloud your judgment and lead to decisions made in haste, without all the information you need to be truly informed about your options and their consequences. Even though others may have had a particular experience or outcome, it doesn't mean that you will too.

Second, it is important to replace fear with knowledge, and ultimately with wisdom. Many of the things you fear about your diagnosis or treatment may simply not be true. Your physician should offer information about your illness, your condition, and the anticipated benefits of therapy. He or she should also explain the possible side effects that are part of many cancer treatments, even though many of them are much less debilitating than they were just a few years ago. You should also have a clear understanding of all your options for different kinds of treatment. If real data about your condition suggests that a particular therapy can have clearly defined benefits, you should strongly consider going ahead with it. Finally, attention must also be given to the mental, emotional, and spiritual aspects of your well-being. Later in this chapter (on page 72) you will find a very effective five-step process to help you make decisions about your treatment.

Third, the unique nature of each patient—not just the specificity of your diagnosis but your essential individuality as a human being—must be addressed.

Every person responds to treatment differently. What is challenging for one person may be a breeze for another. Attitudes and beliefs can also play a big role in how different individuals approach their care. Many patients, for example, have built their identity around health and nutrition and exercise. They want their cancer treatment to be congruent with the healthy lifestyle they've followed for years. While I wholeheartedly believe in following a healthy lifestyle, that lifestyle did not prevent these patients from getting cancer, and it may not prevent cancer from coming back. Once that point has been made, though, decisions can follow on the basis of patients' personal feelings, combined with an accurate picture of their condition.

3. Patients with unresectable or metastatic cancer

A third group of patients are those whose cancer is not curable by surgery because the tumor is technically unresectable, or has spread from the primary site. When cancer spreads to other locations in the body, it is known as *metastatic cancer*. In some cases the orginal, primary site is never identified. Except in very rare instances, surgery is no longer a meaningful option. Therefore, it is not surprising that most patients with unresectable or metastatic tumors are generally less resistant to beginning chemotherapy or radiation treatment, particularly if there is a recognized benefit they can reasonably expect from their therapy. But here, as at every other stage of the journey, no one should focus only on the strictly clinical elements of cancer care. There are many other things you can do to promote healing in body, mind, heart, and spirit, and we will be discussing these throughout the remainder of this book.

For most patients with cancer, but especially those with metastatic cancer, the illusions of immortality that we all tend to harbor are profoundly shaken. This can be emotionally painful and frightening, but it can also be one of the genuinely illuminating effects of the cancer experience. It is an opportunity to have a transforming experience of yourself and the world you live in. It is a chance to learn and grow in ways that you may never before have imagined. Even if your illness is eventually cured, your experience of cancer can make an enormous difference in how you live each day from now on. It can impact—at the very deepest levels—every aspect of the way you engage life, and how you face death as well.

4. Patients whose cancer has relapsed, or is no longer responding to treatment

When a relapse occurs, and it becomes unlikely that a cure will be achieved, an entirely new set of questions arise. At present, approximately

40 percent of all cancer patients will eventually find themselves in this category.

In addition to the spiritual issues that emerge at this point, concerns like pain management, nutrition, and maintaining everyday quality of life reassert their importance with a new urgency. When you or a loved one has cancer that has relapsed or is no longer responding to treatment, what do you do with yourself and how do you choose to spend the time you have left? The realization that life really will end at some point can bring new meaning to every moment and can open undreamed of possibilities for love and growth. If that sounds sentimental, please be aware that I've made the journey through cancer with thousands of people, including members of my own family. I have seen cancer ignite pain, but I've also seen it kindle love, fulfillment, inspiration, and joy at the deepest levels. While few people are oblivious to the first possibility, it is important that they not ignore the second.

Though the explicit goal may no longer be to cure your cancer, there is still a great deal that can and should be done to enhance your enjoyment and quality of life. It is also important to carefully consider further options that might extend survival as well.

New anticancer drugs and therapies are appearing every day, and advances are being made in entirely new domains of treatment. Newspapers, books, magazines, television, and the Internet provide up-to-the-minute information on these developments. Many late-stage patients and their family members hope that a new experimental treatment will cure their disease. This belief often occurs whether the therapy is being offered at a major, National Cancer Institute–designated cancer center or at an alternative medicine clinic in Europe, Mexico, or the Bahamas. It also occurs even if the therapy is an unproven herbal compound that can be purchased through the mail. Very few late-stage patients, or their family members, understand that only a relatively small percentage of patients will personally benefit in a significant way from experimental or unproven therapies. However, when an experimental therapy is offered at a legitimate cancer center, as part of a legitimate clinical trial, the information gained from the trial can be potentially invaluable for the lives of others, and many patients find this meaningful and comforting. Such a benefit is rarely possible at clinics that offer completely unproven, and often completely irrational, alternative therapies.

As someone who has spent his entire adult life dealing with cancer in a clinical setting, I've found that the true miracles of cancer rarely take the form of drugs, potions, or herbs. More often than not, the true miracles take place in the minds, hearts, and spirits of patients and their families.

CANCER QUESTIONS AND ANSWERS

What is cancer?

As stated earlier, cancer is a broad term that encompasses more than a hundred different diseases. Although varying degrees of difference and similarity exist among these diseases, they share certain fundamental characteristics. All cancers involve abnormal cells that differ in two important ways from other cells in the body.

First, cancer cells divide in an uncontrolled, disordered manner. When this happens, they form tumors that can grow, impinge upon, or even invade adjacent tissues and structures in the body.

Second, cancer cells have the capacity to spread from their original point of origin to other sites, where they can continue to grow. This process is called *metastasis*, and, for most cancers, is what causes the most serious problems for patients.

What causes cancer?

This is one of the most controversial and perplexing areas in our understanding of the disease. Contrary to some popular misconceptions, human beings are not the only species to be afflicted with cancer. Virtually all animal species in addition to mammals, including fish, birds, reptiles, and amphibians, have the potential to develop cancer. Tumors have been documented in all of them.

Nor is cancer solely a product of the Industrial Age. Evidence of tumors has been found in Pleistocene cave bears and dinosaurs from the Cretaceous Age, as well as Egyptian mummies from 3000 B.C. Cancer is even mentioned in one of the world's oldest medical treatises, the Edwin Smith Papyrus, which originated in Egypt between 3000 and 2500 B.C. Here, eight classes of tumors or ulcers of the breast are described that are believed to have been treated with primitive forms of surgery. Even Hippocrates, one of the giants of ancient medicine, wrote extensively about cancer in the fourth century B.C. and postulated about its possible causes.

One of the most remarkable and challenging aspects of cancer is that it arises from cells within our own body that were previously normal.

Current medical science describes the origin of cancer as a sequence of events at the cellular level that culminates in the appearance of cancer cells. The sequence begins with changes in the genetic material of normal cells brought about by so-called cancer initiators. These can include *external* factors, such as cigarette smoke, exposure to other carcinogenic chemicals, exposure to ionizing radiation, or, rarely, viruses, and *internal* factors such as abnormal hormonal activity or inherited genetic abnormalities. One of the effects of these initiating factors is to activate certain cancer-causing genes, called *oncogenes*. Just as important, initiating factors can also cause other genes that suppress the development of cancer, called *tumor-suppressor genes*, to become inactive. When the normally fine-tuned balance of activity between oncogenes and tumor-suppressor genes has been disrupted, cancer cells can begin to grow. Once cancer development has been initiated, it can be furthered by the presence of a variety of cancer promoters, including alcohol and a high-fat diet.

Since the discovery of oncogenes in the 1970s, a challenging philosophical question has been raised: Why do human beings have genes in their DNA that can influence the development of cancer? The answer is still unknown. One theory proposed is that—under normal circumstances—these genes may play an important role in the regulation of development of the human embryo. It is when these genes become altered in some way, or are inappropriately activated or overactivated, that they lead to abnormal cell growth and multiplication, which can eventually result in cancer.

While it is tempting to attribute the cause of cancer to events or substances in the external world, or to internal physiologic or genetic changes, an important distinction has to be made between the true *cause* of cancer and the *mechanisms* by which cells become cancerous.

For example, while many people who smoke and drink do get cancer, many more do not. Genetic factors have been cited as a possible explanation for this, but inadequately so. Thus, it remains unclear why individuals can have such widely different manifestations of health or disease. Viruses have also been implicated in the origin of some cancers, though rarely and without a complete understanding of exactly how this can occur. Just as with smoking and drinking, it is still unclear why most people infected with certain potentially cancer-causing viruses never get the disease.

Scientists generally postulate that the difference between individuals will be found in specific deficits or changes in their immune function, or in other constitutional factors. However, the nature of the specific differences in immune function or constitution from one individual to another are still poorly understood.

In recent years, a great deal of attention has been focused on the fact that some people have cancer that appears to run in their families. These inherited predispositions have led to a great deal of research on the possible specific inherited genes that might be causing the problem, such as the *BRCA1* and *BRCA2* genes in breast cancer. While we now understand much more about these genes and the role they may play in the development of cancer in certain individuals, their role in the development of cancer as a whole remains far from clear.

Another area of great interest has to do with the role of the immune system in preventing cancer from appearing, or spreading, in different individuals, whether or not they are infected with certain viruses or exposed to potentially cancer-causing substances. Some scientists postulate that cancer cells—which are known to spontaneously appear in the body on a microscopic level—only rarely grow into full-blown tumors because they are cleared away by scavenger cells of the immune system. This idea is the so-called *immune surveillance theory,* which has found its way, in various forms, into the public eye. Unfortunately, this theory—which remains controversial—has led many people to assume that they got cancer simply because their "immune system is weak." Even more unfortunately, this notion leads many individuals with cancer to mistakenly believe that all they have to do is "boost their immune system" with herbs, mushrooms, vitamins, or other supplements and their cancer will go away. If only it were so simple!

Despite clear evidence that in some instances dysfunction of the immune system is related to the development of cancer, this is by no means a universal phenomenon. Many people with completely normal, functioning immune systems develop cancer. And many more patients with damaged immune systems do not develop cancer. Boosting the immune system of cancer patients with simple methods like herbs and vitamins—or with aggressive methods such as alpha-interferon or interleukin—has not yet proved to be a reliable or effective form of treatment.

One of the major reasons for this has to do with the nature of cancer cells themselves. Since they arise within our own bodies, from our own previously normal cells, it is often hard for the immune system to tell the difference between a normal cell and a cancer cell. Unless the immune cells can accurately identify and distinguish exactly which cells to kill—which is, once again, often hard to do—"boosting" the immune system even to superhuman levels will not help.

Ironically, this same ambiguous quality of cancer cells is one of the things that so often limits the effectiveness of chemotherapy and radiation. The cancer cells often retain so many of the characteristics of their normal progenitor cells that it is very difficult to kill them all without also causing unacceptable damage to normal cells and tissues of the body.

A final important point to mention in this discussion is that cancer has long been thought of as a disease of the elderly. This is because the risk of developing cancer has always increased significantly after the age of fifty. A majority of cancers occur in people over the age of sixty-five, although it is also true that more younger people are being diagnosed with cancer in recent years than ever before. The reasons for this trend are not entirely clear. It seems likely that dietary and environmental factors may be contributing to this phenomenon. As to why cancer still occurs most commonly in the elderly, the answer also remains unclear. One theory postulates diminished immune function, with decreased "immune surveillance" as a significant cause. More recent scientific discoveries suggest other possible contributing factors, including one or more abnormalities in the cells' ability to regulate their own normal life cycle.

There is no question that modern science will continue the search for a deeper understanding of the cellular, molecular, and genetic changes that lead to the development of cancer in humans. And there is no doubt that as scientific tools and technologies progress, newer and more powerful insights will emerge. But for now, a definitive cause of cancer has not been established.

How does cancer harm the body?

As cancer cells reproduce, they can form larger and larger tumors, which may displace normal tissue. The displacement of normal tissue can cause organs to function improperly or to stop functioning altogether. For example, a collection of cancer cells within the liver may initially form small nodules that can increase in number and size. If untreated, these can eventually overwhelm the liver, leading to liver failure and possibly even death. Similar events can occur in virtually every organ and system of the body. When this occurs in the lung, it can cause obstruction of a person's airway, along with cough, pain, or shortness of breath. When it occurs in the colon, it can cause obstruction of the bowel, resulting in abdominal pain and bloating.

When these kinds of obstructions occur, not only is the organ's ability to function impaired, but severe infections can also develop. Bulky tumors can themselves also serve as hiding places for bacteria, be inaccessible to antibiotics, and lead to infections.

Sometimes cancer cells infiltrate important lymph node regions of the body and cause obstruction of the lymphatic channels. When this occurs, the normal flow of lymph fluid can be impaired, and fluid collections can build up around the lungs or heart *(pleural* or *pericardial effusions),* in the abdomen *(ascites),* or in the extremities *(edema).*

Tumors can also invade other structures surrounding their site of origin and cause additional problems, including bleeding, ulcer formation, and pain.

Many types of cancer cells secrete chemicals that can cause a variety of metabolic problems in the body, often called *paraneoplastic phenomena.* Since cancer cells derive from normal cells, these chemicals are usually normal proteins that are now being produced in either excessive quantities or in an inappropriate manner. A common consequence of this phenomenon is the dramatic loss of appetite *(anorexia)* and weight loss *(cachexia)* that some cancer patients experience. Other common manifestations include significant elevations in blood calcium levels *(hypercalcemia)*, abnormalities in blood sodium levels *(hyponatremia)*, nerve damage *(neuropathy)*, and severe muscle weakness *(myopathy)*.

Some cancers also secrete chemicals that interfere with the blood in such a way as to cause blood clots to form. This is commonly called *Trousseau's syndrome*, or a *hypercoagulable disorder*.

Despite the numerous problems and challenges that the original, primary tumor can cause, it is rarely the direct cause of death. By a sequence of extraordinarily complex molecular and cellular processes, cancer cells can invade into and spread through the circulatory or lymphatic systems and form new tumors in multiple locations in the body. This is the most serious aspect of cancer, and the one that causes the most problems for patients and oncologists alike. Physicians use the verb *metastasize* to denote the spread of cancer cells. When a patient's cancer is present in more than one site, the patient is said to have *metastatic disease*.

Why is metastatic cancer so difficult to control?

In cancer treatment, a basic distinction is made between cancers that are curable by surgery and those that are not. In general, when a cancer metastasizes from its primary site, it takes root in one or more new sites. Unfortunately, the location of all of these sites may not be detectable by even the most sophisticated diagnostic procedures, including blood tests, X-rays, bone scans, CT scans, or MRI scans. Since metastases usually involve multiple sites in the body, it is almost always impossible to surgically remove them all. Furthermore, other microscopic sites of disease that are not yet detectable can eventually appear as well. For these reasons, surgery by itself only rarely cures patients who have cancer that has spread to other sites.

When a cancer spreads, it retains much of its original identity—regardless of its new location. Thus, prostate cancer that has spread to the bones is not bone cancer, but *bone metastases of prostate cancer*. Similarly, breast cancer that has spread to the lungs is not lung cancer, but *lung metastases of breast cancer*. Cancer cells that have spread to other locations in the body will often form new tumors in these locations. And since these can rarely be removed surgically, other forms of therapy are generally required, such as chemotherapy or radiation. Here, carefully determining the primary cell of origin of the metastatic tumor is critically important in deciding which kind of chemotherapy, or what dose of radiation, will be required.

One of the most fundamental challenges in oncology is the difficulty in eradicating metastases from the body once they have developed. Once again, a primary reason for this is that cancer cells, though different from normal cells in a number of important ways, are in many other important ways not different enough. Thus, conventional treatments such as chemotherapy or radiation that are used to kill cancer cells often damage or kill many other normal cells in the body at the same time. This is what causes many of the most severe side effects that are associated with conventional treatments. Furthermore, as powerful as conventional treatments are, they are often not powerful or effective enough to eradicate every last cancer cell, so the cancer can eventually grow back.

What are the main groups of cancer?

The overwhelming majority of cancers can be broken down into three main groups: *carcinomas, sarcomas,* and *leukemias/lymphomas.*

The first group, carcinomas, are by far the most common forms of cancer. Carcinoma, meaning "cancerous growth," was introduced into the Latin language by the Roman physician Aurelius Celsus, around A.D. 25–50. He derived the word from the Greek *karkinoma,* meaning "crab," which Hippocrates had first used to describe the condition around 400 B.C. The group of cancers called carcinomas arise principally in the gland-forming cells found in virtually all the organs of the body.

The second group of cancers arise from the body's bone and connective tissues. These are called sarcomas, which is the term the Roman physician Galen first used to describe fleshy tumors, around A.D. 200. Sarcomas are much less common than carcinomas, but there are still many different kinds of sarcomas.

One of the hallmarks of carcinomas and sarcomas, which oncologists refer to as the "solid tumors," is that they usually form discrete masses that can often be surgically removed if discovered early enough.

The third major group of cancers are the leukemias and lymphomas. These arise from the blood and lymph-forming cells of the body, including the bone marrow and lymph nodes. Surgery is almost never an option in these cancers, because they rarely form discrete, solid masses that can be resected.

While these three groups do not account for all cancers, they constitute the vast majority.

How do oncologists describe a patient's particular type of cancer?

A number of features are always assessed when oncologists evaluate a particular patient's cancer. Three of the most important features are the specific *type* of tumor, its *grade,* and the cancer *stage.* These features play a very important role in determining what kind of treatment will be recommended. They can also help predict what kind of response patients might expect from their specific therapy, as well as their prognosis.

TUMOR TYPE. The vast majority of cancers can be classified under the three major groups described above (carcinomas, sarcomas, and leukemias/lymphomas). Within each of these three groups, or classes, of cancer, one finds a large number of specific *types.*

The specific type of cancer corresponds directly to the specific kind of cell from which it has arisen. Type is determined by analyzing a biopsy specimen taken from the tumor. The analysis is usually performed by a specialized physician, called a pathologist. The pathologist will look at the tissue under a microscope and scrutinize its appearance to determine—as best as possible—the specific kind of cell or tissue from which the tumor arose.

For example, a large number of different kinds of cancers arise from gland-forming cells that occur in the various organs of the body—the lungs, esophagus, stomach, pancreas, liver, colon, breast, and prostate, among others. Gland-forming cells perform a variety of functions that specifically define the organ. The gland-forming cells in the colon, for instance, secrete various lubricating molecules and also absorb fluids and nutrients. When the gland-forming cells become cancerous in a particular organ, a carcinoma is said to have occurred in that organ. Specifically, when a gland cell becomes cancerous it is called an *adenocarcinoma*. If cancer arises in the gland-forming cells of the esophagus, it is called an *adenocarcinoma of the esophagus*. If it arises from gland-forming cells of the prostate, it is called an *adenocarcinoma of the prostate*.

Other kinds of cells are found in the various organs and tissues of the body. The esophagus has cells in its inner lining that are called *squamous cells*. When these become malignant and form a tumor, it is referred to as a *squamous cell carcinoma*. Another example is found in the bladder, which has *transitional cells*. When these become malignant, they are referred to as a *transitional cell carcinoma*.

The majority of breast cancers arise from specialized cells which make up the milk ducts. When these cancers invade through the milk ducts they are called *infiltrating ductal carcinoma*. Approximately 70 percent of all breast cancers are of this type. Another, much less common form of breast cancer arises from tissues called breast lobules, which produce milk. When cancer of this type invades through the lobule they are called *infiltrating lobular carcinoma*.

Two other important types of breast cancer are distinguished by their tendency to grow in place without invading into deeper tissues; these are called *in situ carcinomas*. When these arise from duct cells they are called *ductal carcinoma in situ* (DCIS, or sometimes, *intraductal carcinoma*). When they arise from lobular cells they are called *lobular carcinoma in situ* (LCIS, or sometimes, *intralobular carcinoma*). A major factor in how these are treated involves their potential to develop into full-blown invasive cancer.

By carefully identifying exactly which cell a tumor has arisen from, along with a variety of other features, doctors and scientists have learned to categorize the different types of cancer more precisely. Newer and more sophisticated tools and technologies are being developed that allow distinctions between cells to be made at finer and finer levels. As this occurs, new types and forms of cancers are being described that were not recognized before, and this process will also undoubtedly continue in the future.

TUMOR GRADE. Once the pathologist has defined the specific type of cancer involved, the next step is to determine its *grade*. The grade of a tumor is an indication or reflection of how aggressive it is. The grade is primarily determined by a further analysis of the tumor's specific appearance under the microscope.

For example, cancer cells that are similar in appearance to their normal cell of origin are likely to behave in a less aggressive way and are generally classified as *low-grade*. Cancer cells that appear significantly different compared with their normal cell of origin are more likely to behave in a more aggressive manner and are generally classified as *high-grade*. These kinds of cancer cells often have bizarre distinguishing features that make them relatively easy for a pathologist to identify under the microscope. Cancer cells that are intermediate in appearance, and often in their clinical behavior as well, are referred to as *intermediate-grade*.

An individual with a high-grade adenocarcinoma of the prostate will likely have a significantly different clinical course than another individual with a low-grade adenocarcinoma of the prostate. Similarly, the issues involved in treating a woman with a high-grade infiltrating ductal carcinoma of the breast are potentially quite different than for a woman with a low-grade infiltrating ductal carcinoma of the breast.

TUMOR STAGE. This is often one of the most important factors in determining the kind of treatment that will be recommended for a specific cancer, as well as a patient's prognosis.

Tumor stage is actually a representation or description of how far a cancer has spread in the body. In the majority of cases, cancers are described as occurring in one of four different stages.

Stage I tumors, in general, are still localized to the area in which they were discovered. Thus, they are tumors that have not spread.

Stage II tumors, in general, have spread only to the immediately surrounding tissues.

Stage III tumors, in general, have spread a bit farther than Stage II tumors, and often involve nearby lymph nodes.

Stage IV tumors are those that have spread widely, including to other organs.

A variety of different staging systems have been used by oncologists to describe the extent of spread of different cancers. Most oncologists are familiar with most of the different staging systems and routinely use them interchangeably. For example, it is still common for many doctors to refer to the "Duke's" staging system of colon cancer. Another example involves small-cell lung cancer, which is still commonly described in clinical practice as being either "limited" or "extensive" stage.

But the most widely utilized and internationally recognized staging system is called the TNM staging system. Here, the *T* refers to the size of the primary *tumor; N* refers to whether or not the lymph *nodes* are involved with the tumor; and *M* refers to whether or not the cancer has *metastasized* to other organs or tissues.

Regardless of the staging system used, all of them describe the same basic clinical features of the specific cancer, including—most important—the extent to which it has spread. In all of the staging systems, including the TNM system, the higher the stage of the cancer, the more widely it has spread.

Finally, several other factors are often important in the characterization and treatment planning of cancer. One well-known factor, the *hormone receptor status,* is involved in the assessment and treatment of breast cancer. This refers to the presence or absence of estrogen receptors (ER) and progesterone receptors (PR) in the breast cancer cells. The reason this is so important in a particular woman's breast cancer is that tumor cells in which these receptors are absent often behave more aggressively than when they are present. This may influence treatment recommendations as well as prognosis.

Another feature of cancer cells that has been gaining attention in recent years is called *antigen expression.* Antigens are special proteins found on tumor cell surfaces that help distinguish them from normal cells. For example—once again in breast cancer—tumors that express more than the usual amount of the *HER-2/neu* antigen have important characteristics that can greatly influence treatment recommendations and prognosis. In recent years, antigen expression has also led to a greater understanding of the origin of many of the different types of lymphoma and can influence treatment recommendations as well.

Finally, another significant area of interest and research in oncology has focused on specific gene abnormalities, which are being found with increasing frequency in a wide variety of cancers. Understanding of these is now beginning to influence clinical management of different cancers, such as bladder and colon cancer, among others. These are often found to have characteristic abnormalities involving the well-known tumor-suppressor gene *p53*. Similarly, specific abnormalities in the well-known breast cancer genes *BRCA1* and *BRCA2* are now suspected to play a role in how individual breast cancers behave clinically.

What are tumor markers?

Cancer cells sometimes secrete specialized proteins into the bloodstream that can serve as a marker, or indicator, of tumor growth. These are called *tumor markers,* and they can be specifically associated with a particular type of cancer. Sometimes the same tumor marker can be secreted by a variety of different cancers. In other instances, identical proteins can be secreted by normal tissues but usually in much lower amounts.

Not all cancers secrete tumor markers into the bloodstream, but when they do, they can be very helpful in early detection of cancer, monitoring response to treatment, or identifying relapses. In general, when concentrations of a specific tumor marker are found to be significantly elevated, the likelihood is increased that cancer is present. Very often, the blood levels of the marker will fall in response to successful treatment, or not fall if the treatment is not working well. If the marker falls to a very low level after successful cancer treatment, its subsequent rise can indicate that the cancer cells are once again growing—even before any specific symptoms appear.

The most well-known tumor marker today is the PSA, which stands for *prostate specific antigen.* The PSA is a highly specific protein that is secreted only by cells of the prostate gland. It is one of the most widely utilized screening tests for cancer, and will be discussed in greater detail in the section on prostate cancer on page 59. Another well-known tumor marker in use today is the CA 125, which is important in the diagnosis of ovarian cancer, as well as monitoring its response to treatment. Other clinically useful tumor markers include the CEA (*carcinoembryonic antigen*, for colon cancer), CA 15-3 (for breast cancer), CA 19-9 (for pancreas cancer), AFP (*alpha-fetoprotein*, for liver cancer and testicular cancer), and beta-HCG (for testicular cancer).

Research is currently under way on a wide array of newer and more useful tumor markers. These may prove helpful in a variety of ways, including selecting specific treatments and predicting responses to them with much greater precision than ever before.

What are the forms of cancer treatment?

Currently surgery, chemotherapy, and radiation are the three principal categories of cancer treatment. As research continues, immunotherapy, tumor vaccines, and a variety of gene therapies are gaining increased attention.

Surgery is by far the oldest form of treatment for cancer, and it remains the most widely used form today. It is still one of the most effective treatments for a variety of different cancers—particularly when they have not yet spread to other parts of the body. Despite the skill of the surgeons, as well as ingenious advances in the operations themselves, surgery is still essentially akin to pulling weeds out of a garden. It does not deal with what caused the weeds in the first place or address how to prevent them in the future. Yet half of all cancer cures result from surgery, so its importance can hardly be overstated.

The standard practice in cancer surgery has been to remove the tumor itself and as much of the surrounding tissue as possible to prevent the tumor from spreading or growing back. In recent years, the trend has been toward less aggressive surgeries. Medicine is learning that in dealing with cancer more is not necessarily better. The best-known example of this is the replacement of *radical mastectomy* for breast cancer (removal of the entire breast as well as the underlying muscle and tissue) with *modified radical mastectomy* (removal of most of the breast tissue and only a limited amount of underlying tissue). Over the last two decades this trend has been advanced further by *lumpectomy* (removal of just the breast tumor itself, with only a small amount of surrounding tissue) followed by radiation.

Another form of "downsizing" in breast cancer surgery that has gained attention in recent years involves the use of a new technique called *sentinel lymph node biopsy*. Here, surgeons are able to identify and remove just one or two of a patient's axillary lymph nodes, rather than multiple lymph nodes as has been the standard practice, and still obtain the information necessary for prognosis and treatment recommendations.

In contrast to this trend, as surgical techniques continue to advance, many patients with lung and other cancers that were previously considered inoperable are now being successfully treated with more extensive surgeries.

Radiation is also an important treatment modality in cancer care. Its beneficial effects are generally restricted to a specific area of the body where the radiation is focused. In this way, radiation is similar to surgery in that its potential to cure is generally limited to cancers that have not spread to other sites. Radiation occasionally can be just as effective as surgery, while often being much less disfiguring.

Certain types of cancer are very amenable to radiation, such as anal cancer and tumors of the head and neck. Radiation is also effective for certain types of lung cancer, prostate cancer, cervical cancer, tumors of the bone, and lymphomas. For some malignancies such as inoperable brain tumors, it may be the only treatment available. But very often radiation is one element in an overall treatment plan that also includes chemotherapy and/or surgery. It may be used prior to surgery—to shrink a tumor—or after surgery to prevent the regrowth of any remaining tumor cells.

Radiation is believed to cause genetic damage to cancer cells, which cannot easily repair themselves. In contrast, normal tissues that are exposed to radiation are generally better able to repair themselves and heal. That is why radiation can be administered without completely destroying the area surrounding the tumor.

Today radiation therapy is applied using extremely sophisticated techniques, often guided by advanced computer programs, which can focus the radiation beam to a small area that is composed predominantly of tumor cells. Furthermore, in recent years significant advances have been made in the implantation of radioactive materials directly into tumors, called *brachytherapy* or *seed implants*. These techniques are most commonly used in prostate and cervical cancer. They are also now being utilized in breast and lung cancers as well.

A specialized new form of radiation therapy is called *gamma-knife radiosurgery*. This is used predominantly to treat small brain tumors that are inaccessible to conventional surgery.

Chemotherapy is the third element in the standard approach to cancer treatment. It is the youngest of the three modalities, with origins as recent as the 1940s.

Although a certain amount of controversy surrounds chemotherapy in the popular literature on cancer, it is not controversial in the minds of practicing oncologists. In fact, chemotherapy is the foundation of treatment for a very large number of cancer patients. Despite its obvious limitations, when used with great care and skill its benefits are unmistakable, and can be extraordinary.

Different anticancer medicines work in different ways, but all ultimately work by interfering in some way with the division and replication process of cancer cells. Some of the older drugs, such as melphalan (Alkeran), cyclophosphamide (Cytoxan), doxorubicin (Adriamycin), and cisplatin (Platinol) cause the destruction of malignant cells through direct damage to the cell's genetic material, the DNA. Others, such as fluorouracil (5-FU), disrupt cancer cells' ability to replicate by inserting unusable material into the DNA. Several drugs that are derived from plants, notably vincristine (Oncovin), vinblastine (Velban), paclitaxel (Taxol), and docetaxel (Taxotere) interfere in unique ways with specialized proteins within cells that are important for cell division.

Steroid medications such as prednisone (Deltasone) and dexamethasone (Decadron) are also sometimes used in the treatment of cancer. They are particularly toxic to lymphoid cells, in ways that are not entirely clear. Hormones are sometimes used in cancer treatment as well. They suppress the growth of tumors by blocking certain hormone receptors inside the cancer cells, especially in cancer of the breast or prostate.

Chemotherapy has contributed to many extraordinary advances in cancer treatment, especially over the last twenty-five years. However, it remains saddled with three fundamental limitations: side effects, eventual drug resistance by cancer cells, and the inability to reach every cancer cell in the body. Let's deal with each of these directly:

1. SIDE EFFECTS OF CHEMOTHERAPY. These are legion, and well known: fatigue, nausea, vomiting, diarrhea, hair loss, suppression of the bone marrow, nerve damage, kidney damage, loss of appetite, and mouth sores are some of the most common. The primary reason for these side effects is that chemotherapy drugs generally kill cancer cells more effectively when they are dividing rapidly than when they are not. Unfortunately, they also kill normal cells in the body that are also dividing rapidly, such as those found lining the gastrointestinal tract, in hair follicles, and in the bone marrow. It is damage to these normal tissues that usually accounts for the majority of the side effects encountered with chemotherapy.

It is important to recognize that not all patients will suffer from these side effects. Some will experience a number of them, to varying degrees—and others will experience none at all. The side effects also vary with the specific drug being used, the interval of time between treatments, the specific dosage, and the nutritional status and overall condition of the patient.

Fortunately, oncologists are able to give chemotherapy in a manner that minimizes side effects, while still deriving maximum benefit from the drugs. Many new chemotherapy drugs have significantly fewer side effects than older ones and many other medications have been released in recent years that can minimize, if not eliminate outright, a number of the side effects previously associated with chemotherapy.

2. DRUG RESISTANCE. Cancer cells can sometimes have very devious and efficient ways of resisting the effects of chemotherapy, known as *drug resistance*. Over the years, oncologists have employed a number of

different strategies to try to overcome this problem, with only limited success. Another aspect of the problem involves the fact that cancer cells may sometimes become resistant to chemotherapy drugs even if they initially responded to them very well. This is one of the reasons why it can be so hard to actually cure cancer—especially solid tumors—with chemotherapy. If one single cancer cell is not killed by the therapy, it can grow back and cause more problems.

3. CHEMOTHERAPY'S INABILITY TO REACH EVERY CANCER CELL IN THE BODY. This occurs in two major ways. First, some tumors grow so large that blood vessels no longer carry blood to their deepest, innermost regions. Since chemotherapy is carried in the blood, it sometimes can't reach all of the cancer cells that are buried deep inside the tumor. When this happens, those cancer cells survive and can continue to grow, spread to other sites in the body, and develop more resistance to chemotherapy, as described above.

A second way this problem occurs involves what are called *tumor sanctuaries.* These are special areas of the body that are naturally protected from the effects of drugs and toxins in order to keep us well. The two most important areas that are considered to be tumor sanctuaries are the testes and the brain. When cancer cells are found in these organs it is hard for the chemotherapy drugs to reach them, and cancer will often regrow there if not treated with some other means, such as surgery or radiation.

How are chemotherapy drugs administered?

Chemotherapy drugs are administered in a variety of ways, but usually via an intravenous infusion or oral tablet. The intravenous infusions can range in duration from a few minutes, to a few hours, to many days continuously—depending on the drug and the kind of cancer being treated. Hormone therapies are usually administered by tablet, muscular injection, or by a skin patch.

Chemotherapy today is very different from five years ago, to say nothing of twenty-five years ago. One goal of *The Journey Through Cancer* is to dispel the common perception of chemotherapy as a toxic, reprehensible abuse of patients by uncaring physicians. In the 1970s and 1980s the number and efficacy of chemotherapy drugs was limited. But in the last decade new drugs have appeared that are significantly more effective, and in many instances much less toxic.

If there is a real problem with chemotherapy, it is often not in the drugs but in the level of consciousness, skill, and attentiveness with which they are administered. Successful use of these medications demands a real commitment to caring for the patients who receive them. Two patients may take the same dose of the same drug, but the manner in which it is given—the environment, the care with which it is administered, the fears and expectations of the patient, and his or her overall physical status—are all very important factors in influencing the patient's experience. Meticulous follow-up is also extremely important. A doctor who fails to closely monitor a chemotherapy patient is like a driver who takes his eyes off the road. It only takes a split second for a serious accident to occur.

What are the most common forms of cancer?

By far, the most common form of cancer in America is skin cancer, including basal cell and squamous cell carcinomas. The overwhelming majority of these skin cancers are noninvasive, however, and are easily cured by surgery. Melanoma is another form of skin cancer that has been increasing in incidence in recent years. While this form of skin cancer can be invasive and deadly, it is still relatively uncommon, with about 44,000 cases in 1999.

Other than skin cancer, cancers of the prostate, breast, lung, and colon account for the majority of invasive cancer diagnoses in the United States. Each of these diseases has a number of subtypes, and their characteristics vary among individual patients.

In 1999, these four major types of cancer accounted for more than 50 percent of all invasive cancer cases in the United States: prostate (179,000 cases); breast (176,000 cases); lung (172,000 cases); and colorectal (130,000 cases)—a total of approximately 657,000 cases, out of approximately 1.2 million cases of invasive cancer overall. After colorectal cancer, the most common types of cancer are lymphoma (64,000 cases), bladder cancer (54,000 cases), melanoma (44,000 cases), uterine cancer (37,000 cases), kidney cancer (30,000 cases), leukemias (30,000 cases), pancreas cancer (28,000 cases), and ovarian cancer (25,000 cases).

In the pages that follow, some of the important issues in prostate cancer (below), breast cancer (page 62), lung cancer (page 64), colon cancer (page 66), ovarian cancer (page 67), and lymphoma (page 67) will be addressed in greater detail.

What are the important issues in prostate cancer?

Prostate cancer arises from gland-forming cells of the prostate gland—a walnut-sized organ adjacent to the urinary bladder in men. The specific cause, or causes, of prostate cancer remain unknown, though there are several well-recognized risk factors for developing the disease.

By far, as with most cancers, the most well-established risk factor is age. Diagnosis of prostate cancer is rare before age fifty, but thereafter incidence as well as mortality rates increase dramatically—prostate cancer is actually a common disease in elderly men. Estimates from different studies suggest that undetected prostate cancer may be present in as many as 43 percent of men by age eighty. In many of these men, however, the disease will never become clinically significant. This important fact has contributed greatly to the current debate about the best way to manage prostate cancer, particularly in elderly men.

A strong family history of prostate cancer can increase a man's risk of developing the disease by a factor of two. Another well-accepted risk factor is race. The incidence of prostate cancer in African-American men is higher than among Caucasian men. African-American men also tend to have more aggressive tumors and a higher mortality from the disease. For reasons that are not yet clear, prostate cancer is less common in Asian men, and rarest of all in Chinese men. Dietary factors have also been implicated in the risk of developing prostate cancer, including high intake of animal fat and deficiency of vitamin D. However, these risks are still less well defined compared with other risk factors, and remain somewhat controversial.

Widespread screening for prostate cancer began in earnest in the mid-1980s, utilizing both digital rectal examination of the prostate gland

and the serum PSA test. (PSA stands for *prostate-specific antigen*, as described earlier.) By early 1997, data collected from numerous clinical studies suggested that, since prostate cancer screening could lead to earlier detection, it might also lead to decreased mortality. This has not been conclusively proven, and a great deal of controversy remains regarding the overall benefits of widespread screening for prostate cancer.

False positive screening tests can lead to unnecessary biopsies and other costly and/or uncomfortable diagnostic studies. Annual screening of millions of men without a proven reduction in mortality will add further costs to a society and a health care system that are already heavily burdened. In light of these controversies, additional studies are under way to define the benefits of widespread screening for prostate cancer.

In the meantime, the American Cancer Society has issued the following recommendations.

Beginning at age fifty, men who have a life expectancy of at least ten years should undergo an annual digital rectal examination of the prostate gland and a serum PSA test.

Normal as well as cancerous prostate cells produce and secrete PSA into the bloodstream, but cancerous prostate cells do so much more readily than normal prostate cells. In the absence of prostate cancer, the blood level of PSA is usually less than 4 nanograms per milliliter (ng/ml). When the level of PSA in the blood increases above 4 ng/ml, the likelihood of cancer being present increases.

It is important to remember that not all men with PSA levels above 4 ng/ml will have prostate cancer. Other benign conditions can cause an elevation of the PSA level without cancer being present, including benign prostatic hypertrophy (BPH) or prostatitis (inflammation of the prostate gland, usually caused by infection). Also, a man with a PSA level of less than 4 ng/ml can occasionally have prostate cancer, particularly if the tumor is poorly differentiated, but this is not common.

Screening should begin at a younger age—for example, forty-five—for men who are in a high-risk group for developing prostate cancer. Examples of this group include men with a strong family history of prostate cancer and African-American men.

Digital rectal examination of the prostate gland should be performed by health care professionals who are skilled in the procedure and experienced in recognizing subtle abnormalities of the gland that might suggest the presence of cancer.

As with almost all other forms of cancer, prostate cancer has a wide spectrum of presentations, and the issues involved in treatment vary widely as well. Some of the major forms of treatment that are currently used for nonmetastatic tumors are:

- *Radical prostatectomy,* or surgical removal of the prostate gland, along with regional lymph nodes
- *Nerve-sparing prostatectomy,* which can greatly reduce some of the most troubling long-term side effects of prostatectomy
- *External beam radiation therapy,* which involves radiation targeted at the tumor
- *Seed implant radiation therapy,* in which small radioactive "seeds" are implanted directly into the prostate gland of patients, usually under ultrasound guidance
- *Cryosurgery,* which involves inserting probes containing liquid nitrogen directly into the prostate gland, in order to freeze and kill the cancerous cells
- *Combination therapy,* in which patients are treated with hormone therapy followed by radiation or surgery
- *"Watchful waiting,"* in which patients are followed prospectively by their physician and monitored closely for any signs of progression of their disease before any specific treatment is initiated.

When prostate cancer has spread to other parts of the body, the initial treatment usually involves some form of hormone therapy. In recent years, various kinds of chemotherapy drugs have also been used, particularly in patients whose cancer has become resistant to hormone treatments. When this occurs, the patient is said to have *hormone refractory disease.*

Over the last decade prostate cancer has become an enormous public health issue in the United States, and its impact in our culture will undoubtedly be felt for years to come. With increased awareness of this disease, however, and with continued advances in diagnosis and treatment, the prognosis of men who are diagnosed with prostate cancer should continue to improve significantly in the future.

What are the important issues in breast cancer?

Breast cancer is one of the most readily treatable cancers in humans. It is an area in which new treatment protocols are rapidly appearing and established ones are continuously being revised. There is also no doubt that breast cancer is one of the most controversial and politicized health issues in the United States.

A number of risk factors for breast cancer have been identified. Age is clearly important, as incidence increases significantly in women over fifty. A family history of breast cancer is also associated with a higher predisposition to developing the disease.

Increased exposure to estrogen over many years is believed to heighten a woman's chance of developing breast cancer. This can occur in women who experience early menses or late menopause, who become pregnant for the first time after age thirty or never have children, and who have never breast-fed. Numerous studies have demonstrated a higher risk of breast cancer among women in these groups. It is also believed that alcohol may result in higher estrogen activity, and three large studies have indicated that risk of breast cancer increases with increased alcohol consumption.

Interestingly, exercise has been shown to be helpful in reducing the risk of breast cancer in women. This is presumed to be related to decreased estrogen levels in women who exercise for substantial periods of time, particularly more than four hours per week.

Many attempts have been made over the years to link breast cancer with specific eating habits and to recommend foods that would reduce risk or even "prevent" the appearance of the disease. Although it's tempting to search for these dietary benefits, conclusive evidence has been difficult to establish. At the present time, the role of dietary factors in cancer risk remains hotly debated, although the bulk of available evidence does suggest that eating a plant-based diet provides some protective benefits. Further research may lead to even more specific recommendations for women to follow.

In addition to the shifts in our understanding of specific risk factors for developing breast cancer, the conceptual paradigm of the biology of breast cancer is also changing. Throughout the early years of this century, breast cancer was thought to spread in an organized, predictable manner: beginning with an enlarging mass in the breast, then extending to the axillary lymph nodes before spreading throughout the body. Over the last several decades, however, as our understanding of breast cancer has advanced, it has become recognized that there is often not an orderly progression of the disease. For example, a small tumor in the breast of one woman may have already spread at the time of her diagnosis, while a larger tumor in the breast of another woman may remain localized for a long period of time.

Two significant developments in the treatment of breast cancer have emerged as a result of this new understanding. The first relates to the surgical management of breast cancer, as mentioned earlier in this chapter. Clinical trials have shown that lumpectomy with radiation confers the same survival benefits to many women as mastectomy would, and with much less disfigurement. This controversy extended over several decades, but has now been resolved.

An extension of the evolving role of surgery in breast cancer concerns axillary lymph node dissection, which in a significant percentage of women can lead to debilitating swelling in the arm, known as *lymphedema*. Sentinal lymph node biopsy is advancing in utility and acceptance, and may eventually supplant axillary lymph node dissection entirely, particularly in women with early-stage disease.

The second significant development in the management of breast cancer involves the use of adjuvant chemotherapy. This has now been proven to reduce the risks of recurrence in virtually all women with breast cancer. However, the degree of risk reduction depends upon a number of factors, including the patient's age, the size and grade of the primary tumor, the tumor's hormone receptor status, and the number of lymph nodes involved at the time of diagnosis.

Another controversy surrounds the question of breast cancer screening, particularly in women under the age of fifty. While the PSA test has become a safe and important screening technique for prostate cancer, there is no comparable screening tool for breast cancer. Currently, the methods of detection for breast cancer are still limited to breast self-examination and mammography.

It is clear that mammograms for women over fifty save lives, but do they have similar benefits for younger women? As with prostate cancer, considerable burden on society and the health care system would result from regularly testing millions of additional women with no clear proven benefit—in addition to significant anxiety and inconvenience for the women themselves. These remain hotly debated issues, and women under fifty should speak directly with their physicians about appropriate mammography screening.

Again, breast cancer is one of the most treatable, if not always curable, forms of cancer. It is an area in which new drugs are rapidly appearing, including the anticancer drugs paclitaxel (Taxol), docetaxel (Taxotere), vinorelbine (Navelbine), and capecitabine (Xeloda); hormone therapies like anastrazole (Arimidex) and lotrozole (Femara); and the monoclonal antibody trastuzumab (Herceptin).

New and technically sophisticated treatments, including stem cell transplant, have become widely used. Stem cells are unique cells in the bone marrow that have the ability to develop into all the different kinds of cells found in the blood—red cells, white cells, and platelets. However, recently published studies indicate that the benefits of stem cell transplantation for long-term survival of women with metastatic disease may not be as helpful as many people hoped and believed it would be. Research on this and other complex issues in breast cancer will continue to require time and attention. But there is no question that important progress is taking place.

What are the important issues in lung cancer?

Lung cancer, which was almost unheard of one hundred years ago, is one of the greatest public health travesties ever to befall humankind. This disease could be virtually eliminated if the dissemination of cigarettes were to stop. And if lung cancer were eliminated, 30 percent of all cancer cases in the United States would also be eliminated.

Lung cancer is most often diagnosed when patients present with symptoms such as cough, weight loss, or shortness of breath. Sometimes the diagnosis is made from a chest X-ray done during a routine physical examination or prior to a surgical procedure. As with mammography for younger women, the question of screening for lung cancer with X-rays or sputum cytology has not conclusively been proven to save lives and thus remains controversial. However, an intriguing study published in *The Lancet* in 1999 suggested that screening with CT scans of the chest—which are able to detect lung cancers at a much earlier stage than routine chest X-rays—might lead to improved survival in people who are at high risk.

Until recently, lung cancer was one of the least curable forms of cancer. But the paradigm is shifting in the treatment of lung cancer, particularly in recent years with FDA approval of drugs such as paclitaxel (Taxol), carboplatin (Paraplatin), and gemcitabine (Gemzar). Once unthinkable numbers of people are now living for as long as five years. This is a very significant advance in a disease that was not long ago commonly fatal within six to twelve months. As with most other cancers, a fundamental issue in lung cancer is whether the tumor can be surgically removed at an early stage. When that is the case, five-year survival rates are fairly high.

The disease is divided into two main categories: *small-cell* and *non-small-cell* lung cancer.

Small-cell lung cancer, which accounts for about 25 percent of total cases, has been divided into two subgroups, called *oat cell* and *intermediate cell*, based on their microscopic appearance. The remaining 75 percent of lung cancer cases are of the non-small-cell variety. These occur in three main subgroups, called adenocarcinoma, large-cell carcinoma, and squamous cell carcinoma, based on their cell of origin.

At the time of diagnosis, small-cell lung cancer is much more often disseminated than is true of the other forms. Small-cell lung cancers are also sensitive to radiation and chemotherapy. They respond extremely well, and a significant percentage of limited-stage tumors, and even some advanced-stage ones, can have remarkable—even complete—responses to conventional treatment. Unfortunately, they also have a tendency to recur.

Non-small-cell lung cancers have in the past been more resistant to chemotherapy and radiation. But when treated with the newly available drugs—by themselves, or in combination with radiation or even surgery—the disease can respond more dramatically than ever before, prolonging life in many patients.

Lung cancer is no longer the uniformly dire illness that it was. With early diagnosis and proper treatment, the outlook is now much brighter.

What are the major issues in colon cancer?

A unique feature of colon cancer is that premalignant tissues can be clearly identified and removed in many patients. To take advantage of this fact, screening for colon cancer is very important in higher risk individuals, including people over fifty and those with a strong family history of the disease. When colon cancer is detected early, it is highly curable by surgery. When the tumor has extended through the bowel wall, or spread into local or regional lymph nodes, it is still often curable with surgery followed by adjuvant chemotherapy.

Most colon cancers develop from polyps, which are growths arising from mucous membranes in the wall of the colon. Polyps are common in adults and are usually benign. If they are detected early enough, they can often be removed with a fiber-optic scope (called a sigmoidoscope or colonoscope) on an outpatient basis. If the polyp grows too large surgery may be required. Occasionally, benign polyps can become cancerous and begin to invade the colon wall. In these cases, surgery is usually required and a segment of the colon must be removed as well.

As with other kinds of cancer, treatment decisions for colon cancer are based on staging of the disease in an individual patient. There are several staging systems in use (the Duke's system, the Modified Astler-Coller system, and the TNM staging system), which describe various stages of the illness, from localized to metastatic. In addition to surgery, chemotherapy is an important aspect of colon cancer treatment, especially on an adjuvant basis. New applications of chemotherapy, radiation, and immunotherapy are currently in clinical trials.

What are the major issues in ovarian cancer?

This disease has gained increased attention since the death of the popular actress Gilda Radner in 1989. Today there are roughly 25,000 cases of ovarian cancer annually in the United States. Ovarian cancer has been called "the silent killer" because it can develop and progress with no symptoms whatsoever, until it is finally discovered in an advanced stage. When this occurs, it is often difficult to cure. Screening the general population of women for ovarian cancer remains controversial. However, women who are at high risk for developing the disease may be screened with a pelvic ultrasound and the CA 125 blood test. It is important to be aware that the CA 125 blood test is not entirely reliable, because there are a number of conditions that can cause false positive results. Accurate diagnosis usually requires surgery and a biopsy.

Standard treatment for ovarian cancer includes surgery and chemotherapy. In recent years the drugs Taxol and carboplatin have significantly improved survival rates, allowing many patients to live for years longer than was true in the past.

What are the major issues in lymphoma?

The lymphomas are a diverse group of cancers that arise from various cells of the lymphoid system of the body. They can occur wherever normal lymphocytes are found, including lymph nodes, visceral organs, skin, bones, or even the brain. In general, lymphomas are divided into two main groups, Hodgkin's disease and non-Hodgkin's lymphomas.

Non-Hodgkin's lymphomas (approximately 57,000 cases in 1999) are far more common than Hodgkin's disease (approximately 7,000 cases in 1999). For reasons that are not clear, in recent years non-Hodgkin's lymphomas have been increasing significantly in incidence in the United States and are now the fifth most common cancer in this country.

Historically, a variety of classification systems have been used to define and describe non-Hodgkin's lymphomas. The most commonly used system is called "The Working Formulation." This divides ten major subtypes of non-Hodgkin's lymphomas into low, intermediate, or high-grade groups. In recent years, a new classification system has begun to emerge, called the "REAL Classification System," which is slowly gaining more widespread acceptance.

One of the hallmarks of non-Hodgkin's lymphomas is that they are usually highly responsive to chemotherapy and radiation. However, depending on the stage of the lymphoma, along with its specific grade and subtype, non-Hodgkin's lymphomas can range in behavior from indolent and slow-growing to highly aggressive and lethal. For this reason, it is important for oncologists to know precisely which kind of lymphoma they are dealing with, particularly when formulating a treatment plan. Cure rates for different non-Hodgkin's lymphomas are quite varied, but in general are less than for Hodgkin's disease.

Hodgkin's disease—which was first described in 1832 by the English physician Thomas Hodgkin—has characteristics that are distinct and in many ways quite different from non-Hodgkin's lymphomas. For example, it generally occurs in younger patients and it progresses much more predictably than non-Hodgkin's lymphomas. It is also curable in the majority of cases. In fact, along with testicular cancer, Hodgkin's disease is regarded as one of the most reliably curable forms of cancer.

What is a clinical trial?

As we've discussed, there are many different types of cancer, and within each type there are often many variations. The standard treatment for each kind of cancer represents the culmination of both laboratory research and clinical experience with many patients over long periods of time. Standard treatments, however, are always subject to change based on new information. When a new drug or technique has achieved positive results in laboratory testing, it then becomes available for carefully monitored clinical trials with cancer patients.

Clinical trials are typically designated as Phase I, II, or III. Phase I trials are intended primarily to determine how new treatments affect human patients and specifically what range of doses is safe and acceptable. Because of the risks that may be associated with Phase I trials, they typically only involve patients whose illness is no longer responding to standard treatments. For patients who enroll in Phase I trials, there is usually a small, but real, potential for being helped by the new treatment. There is also the opportunity to advance medical knowledge, which may help others in the future.

Phase II and III trials usually involve larger numbers of participants than Phase I trials. The purpose of Phase II trials is to define more precisely the benefits of new treatments on specific types of cancer. Phase III trials compare new treatments—that were found to be effective in Phase II trials—with previously used standard treatments.

As a cancer patient, you may ask or be asked to participate in a clinical trial. However, you are never required to do so. You will be informed of all the risks and potential benefits of the trial. If you decide to participate you will be asked to sign a document attesting to your informed consent. You can also choose to leave the trial at any time, and this decision will in no way be held against you.

Participating in a Phase III clinical trial does not guarantee that you'll get the new treatment being studied. By a process of random selection, a certain number of patients will receive the new treatment while others will not. In some cases, neither you nor your doctor will know whether you are a member of the treatment group or the control group. These are called "double-blind" studies. However, you will at all times be carefully monitored for your response to treatment and for any potential side effects.

USING EDUCATION AND INFORMATION IN THE DECISION-MAKING PROCESS

In this chapter we have addressed many of the questions that typically rush through the minds of patients upon receiving a cancer diagnosis. Some patients are much less troubled by questions, however, or by a need for detailed, specific answers. They are content to allow their physician, or their family members, to guide a majority of their treatment decisions. For an oncologist, recognizing and responding appropriately to these two broad categories of patients—and everyone in between—requires good judgment and a clear understanding of the role of information in the treatment process.

Even though there is a broad spectrum of interest and need for information among patients and family members, everyone can benefit greatly by understanding the basic facts presented above. Many patients have an endless number of questions, each of which they often believe is a matter of life or death. This desperate hunger for information raises issues that go to the heart of the doctor-patient relationship, as well as the treatment process itself.

Experience has taught me that, in general, patients themselves should decide what information they need or want. They should certainly have all of the information necessary to make truly informed decisions about their care and to understand the effect of their illness and treatment on all areas of their lives.

Unfortunately, many patients often feel that they *do not* have all the information they need or want. Caught in fear or lack of understanding, they complain, "My doctor didn't answer all of my questions," or "My doctor doesn't spend enough time with me." All too often this is true, and their complaints are justified. If you feel this way, express your concerns directly to your physician.

In order to get the answers you want, it is best to be aware of the thoughts and questions that are running through your mind and to put them into words in a way that seems most comfortable. Avoid making any judgments about the questions you want to ask and make it a point to *write your questions down* so you don't forget them.

THE IMPORTANCE OF TRUSTING YOUR GUIDE ON THE JOURNEY THROUGH CANCER

With this in mind, we can return to the issue of trust between doctor and patient from a somewhat different perspective.

Level One of this program is not intended to provide a specific, meticulous answer to every possible question that a patient or family member might have. Rather, it seeks to provide some of the basic information that you and your family need in order to make informed decisions about your care and then to move forward on your healing journey with trust, confidence, and faith in your guide.

As a patient, you must at some point find a way to suspend the unceasing activity of a doubting mind. This is not to suggest that you should abandon thinking or abdicate your sovereign right to know and understand what is happening to you. However, if the doubting mind is left unchecked it can seriously undermine the treatment process.

George Fairfax was someone who seemed to be following such a self-sabotaging path. He was a fifty-one-year-old man with a relatively straightforward type of cancer, and he gave the impression of a deep unwillingness to trust. When I met him, he had already been to the Mayo Clinic in Minnesota, the M. D. Anderson Cancer Center in Houston, and Memorial Sloan-Kettering Cancer Center in New York for consultations about his case. At each of these institutions he was given the same general recommendations for treatment, but he was neither convinced nor satisfied. Now he had come to me for yet another consultation.

Mr. Fairfax was a cyclone of information need. He wanted to know everything about all of the various chemotherapy drugs recommended as part of his treatment. Moreover, he wanted to know about every single possible side effect that could possibly occur, no matter how unlikely. He also wanted to know exactly what I was going to do, *in advance,* to prevent—or at least minimize to the greatest extent possible—all of these possible side effects. He further wanted to know everything about shark cartilage, Essiac tea, vitamins, mineral supplements, antioxidants, and much more.

After a lengthy discussion about all of this, it became clear that his operative impulse was not really a desire to know about cancer or the details of cancer treatment. Instead, he was plagued by a deeply rooted fear of pain, and difficulty in trusting and letting go. As a result, a tremendous amount of valuable time and energy was being diverted into unfulfilling and clinically unproductive channels.

"Mr. Fairfax," I finally said to him, "it is very important that at some point you make a decision to trust someone to guide you in this process. Maybe that person will be me, and, if so, I would be honored to help you.

But if it is not me, then you must find someone else whom you do fully trust. I don't need you to trust and have confidence in me for my sake. It's for *your* sake. If you don't make a decision to fully trust me—or someone else—as your physician, you'll never stop worrying and wondering. You'll burden yourself mentally and emotionally whenever a neighbor, a friend, or a relative tells you about something seen on the Internet, or about a different chemotherapy protocol offered somewhere, or about some new miracle herb or vitamin.

Everyone involved with cancer must ultimately develop the ability to live with uncertainty. Cancer is an area of human experience in which we simply do not have all the answers we want. Caregivers as well as patients have a responsibility to accept the uncertainty that is inevitably part of this journey.

The journey will undoubtedly include unpredictable experiences, and we must recognize that its destination is, in many ways, unknown. By embracing this perspective, no matter what the outcome, you can find love and joy at every step along the way.

How to Make the Most Enlightened Decisions About Your Treatment

Many cancer patients make treatment decisions out of fear—fear of what will happen if they agree to the treatment, or fear of what will happen if they don't. I believe that it is critically important for patients to resolve, here and now, that they will not make treatment-related decisions based on fear. Those decisions—like all decisions in life—are best made when based on entirely different criteria.

The decision-making system outlined here defines the specific criteria that can be extremely helpful for patients and family members on the journey through cancer. It is designed to use with the help of your physicians and other caregivers. For each of the categories, think about the questions in parentheses, then write your thoughts in the space provided or on a separate sheet of paper. After a day or so, look over what you've written and see if your feelings are still the same. If so, you're probably getting close to the decision you truly believe in. If your feelings have changed, write down your new thoughts and give yourself more time to choose the best option. Finally, make sure that you discuss these issues with your physician.

1. **Knowledge and Information** *("Do I really have the knowledge and information I need to make the best decision about my care?" "What does that knowledge and information suggest as the best thing to do in the situation I am facing?")*

_____

_____

_____

_____

_____

2. **Understanding** *("Do I really, truly understand what this knowledge, this information, and all these statistics really mean?"* Often there is a big distinction between *having* information and *understanding* what it means. Ask yourself: *"Do I really understand the implications of choosing this particular treatment?"* Or, *"Do I feel I have a sufficient level of understanding to trust my doctor's recommendation, and feel good about going ahead?"* If you are considering declining a particular treatment, ask yourself: *"Do I really understand the consequences of declining this treatment?" "Do I know and understand what the alternatives are, and what is involved in pursuing them?")*

_____

_____

_____

_____

3. Wisdom (*"What is the wise thing to do?" "What does my deep inner wisdom say to me about these choices?" "What is the wisest choice in terms of accomplishing my most important goals in life?"* For this part of the process, you need to enter deeply into silence and listen for the voice of your inner wisdom. You may wish to be guided in meditation or into a deep state of relaxation in order to hear this inner voice. You must also have clarity about what your goals are. These issues will be addressed in more detail in Chapter 9, Level Six: Life Assessment.)

_____

_____

_____

_____

_____

_____

4. Love and Compassion (You must also ask, *"What is the most loving and compassionate thing to do—for myself and for the people I love and who love me?"* Be aware of the difference between what may seem most loving and compassionate in the short term, as opposed to what may be most loving and compassionate over a longer period of time. Be honest with yourself! This is your life, and your treatment.)

_____

_____

_____

_____

_____

_____

5. Intuition (After all of the previous questions have been answered, it is time for you to tune in to your intuition for additional guidance. This is a part of your unconscious mind that can speak from a place beyond logic or rational thought. This final step should not be taken before the other steps have been completed. The reason for this is that inner voices of fear and doubt can often masquerade as intuition and steer you off-track. Thus, it is important to clear away the voices of fear and doubt by first addressing the questions above.)

_____

_____

_____

_____

_____

5

LEVEL TWO:
PSYCHOSOCIAL SUPPORT

TRUE LISTENING IS LOVE IN ACTION.

—M. SCOTT PECK

Connection with other people lies at the heart of healing. This is true for cancer or any other illness. Though it can take many forms, the need for human connection is as basic as the need for surgery or chemotherapy or any other medical treatment.

Strong scientific evidence now shows that love and support from others translates into better health, not just emotional but physical as well. Multiple prospective studies have confirmed what we might intuitively expect: people with diversified social networks live longer and healthier lives than those who are socially isolated. These health-promoting social ties can take many forms, including marriage, family, friends, neighbors, and colleagues, as well as a variety of social and religious groups.

We now know with certainty that the nervous system, the endocrine system, the digestive system—and indeed all the biological systems of the human body—are inseparably interwoven. While the precise role of stress, anxiety, depression, and other psychological factors in the origin of cancer is still unclear, there is no longer any question about the importance of these factors in influencing a patient's experience of treatment and recovery.

Assessing the impact of psychosocial interventions in the overall care of cancer patients and their families is now a major area of research.

These interventions can take a number of forms, including educational programs and various types of psychological counseling. Perhaps best known, however, are the wide variety of support groups for cancer patients and family members that have gained recognition and acceptance over the past decade.

It is now very clear that support groups *work*. It has been repeatedly shown, for example, that a variety of cancer-support programs can reduce the need for pain medicine, sleeping pills, and medications for depression and anxiety. Patients consistently report improvements in their overall sense of well-being and their sense of control and understanding of their disease. Support groups also give patients the strength and confidence they need to adhere more fully to their treatment plans, which can often have a powerful and positive impact on the course of their illness.

Remarkably, not only do patients report these and other improvements in their quality of life, but *family members report them as well*, even if it was only the patient who participated in the groups.

Support groups can dramatically relieve the overwhelming sense of isolation that is so often experienced by cancer patients. Again and again, patients refer to the isolation they feel when they are diagnosed, even if they are married and have families. The disease causes them to feel cut off from the rest of humanity, separated from everyone in the world who doesn't have cancer. As painful as this is, it can lead patients to isolate themselves even *further*, even from other patients, and this plays into the hands of the disease process. Isolation is both a cause and an effect of depression, and untreated depression can clearly and adversely affect quality of life, immune function, treatment compliance, and even life-expectancy.

On the other hand, when a cancer patient uses the diagnosis for making new connections rather than losing old ones, the experience of the illness changes profoundly. Instead of imposing an enforced isolation, cancer can become a bridge to a larger world. For many patients, support groups are a big part of that positive transition. It is not simply a matter of getting support, but giving it as well. Charlotte Millspaugh, a licensed clinical social worker who leads the support group program at the Geffen Cancer Center, is convinced that participants often gain strength by *providing support to others*, sometimes even more than by receiving it themselves.

For many individuals—including patients, clinicians, and research-ers—an important issue in evaluating psychosocial support is whether it prolongs survival. I believe that focusing on the value of psychosocial support in this way is missing the point, particularly in light of its other significant, and undisputed, benefits. However, several well-known and intriguing studies suggest that psychosocial support may indeed prolong survival times among cancer patients. Although the evidence remains controversial, this research is well worth mentioning.

In 1989, Dr. David Spiegel of Stanford University published the results of a landmark study in the British medical journal *The Lancet* on the effects of a support group for women with metastatic breast cancer. In Dr. Speigel's study, eighty-six women with metastatic breast cancer were randomly assigned to two different groups. Both groups of women received standard medical care for their breast cancer, under the direction of their oncologist. In addition to receiving standard medical care, how-ever, one of the two groups of patients also met once a week for ninety minutes over the course of a year.

The original intent of this study was to assess the effects of the sup-port group intervention on patients' quality of life during the course of their illness. Those women who participated in the support group expe-rienced significantly less anxiety, depression, and pain. They also felt bet-ter able to communicate with their families and their doctors, and enjoyed a greater sense of overall well-being.

Dr. Spiegel had expected these benefits and was gratified to find them. The actual hypothesis of his study, however, had been that psycho-social support and the consequent improvement in quality of life *would not affect* the clinical course of the disease. Dr. Spiegel had been disturbed by reports from patients that they felt they had been "blamed" for their cancer because of their supposedly negative thoughts, or because they had allowed their illness to happen in some other way. As he recounts in his book, *Living Beyond Limits*, Dr. Spiegel believed his research could put to rest once and for all the idea that the right mental attitude had any effect on the course of the disease, by showing that women who partici-pated in a support group lived no longer than those who did not.

Yet, this is exactly the *opposite* of what happened—and no one was more surprised than David Spiegel himself. After ten years of follow-up,

Dr. Spiegel was shocked to discover that the women who had participated in the support group lived 36.6 months, compared with 18.9 months for the women who did not. "In other words," Dr. Spiegel noted, "on average, patients who had been in the experimental treatment program lived *twice as long* from the time they entered the study as did the control patients. This was a difference so significant that statistical analysis was almost unnecessary—all you had to do was look at the curves. And I had been expecting no difference at all!"

The results of this study, which was well-designed and conducted by a respected researcher at a major university medical center, raised quite a stir among oncologists and other cancer researchers. Dr. Spiegel and his team had been careful to examine whether any variables other than participating in the support program might have accounted for the difference in survival between the two groups of women—and none could be found. Could it possibly be true that something as simple as one year of a weekly support group could improve survival so dramatically in people with cancer? For the participants of Dr. Spiegel's study, the answer was an unequivocal *yes*.

Other studies also suggest that psychosocial support for cancer patients may help to prolong life, as well as enhance it.

In 1993, UCLA psychiatrist Dr. Fawzy I. Fawzy and his colleagues published the results of a study in the *Archives of General Psychiatry* involving sixty-eight patients who had undergone standard surgical treatment for malignant melanoma, a potentially deadly form of skin cancer. As with the Spiegel study, Fawzy's patients were divided into two groups. One group of patients had surgery alone. The other patients had the same surgery and also participated in a structured group program lasting ninety minutes a week for six weeks, beginning shortly after their surgery was completed.

At the end of the six-week intervention, patients who had participated in the group reported feeling more vigorous than the patients who had not. At a six-month follow-up evaluation, the differences between the two groups of patients were even more pronounced. Those who had participated in the support program showed significantly lower depression, fatigue, confusion, and mood disturbance, as well as better coping skills, compared with the group who had received surgery alone.

Even more remarkably, at the end of six years of follow-up, Fawzy and his colleagues discovered that patients who had undergone the six-week intervention program had lower recurrence rates and *significantly improved survival.* Specifically, 31 out of 34 patients in the intervention group were alive, compared with 24 of 34 in the surgery-only group. Careful analysis of all possible contributing variables yielded a compelling, unmistakable finding: *the only significant difference between the two groups of patients was the participation by one group in the six-week intervention program.*

In the conclusion of his published article, Dr. Fawzy commented: "Psychiatric interventions that enhance effective coping and reduce affective distress appear to have beneficial effects on survival but are *not* proposed as an alternative or independent treatment for cancer or any other illness or disease. However, the exact nature of this relationship warrants further investigation."

A third provocative study on the importance of social support was undertaken by the Canadian epidemiologist Dr. Elizabeth Maunsell. Her research, which was published in the journal *Cancer* in 1995, involved 224 Canadian women who had undergone surgery for breast cancer that was localized or had spread to regional lymph nodes. Three months after their surgery each of the women underwent an in-depth home interview performed by the same specially trained nurse. The interview included questions on a variety of psychosocial factors, including whether they had confided their feelings or discussed personal problems with one or more persons in the three months following hospitalization. Confidants include spouses, family members, children, friends, neighbors, colleagues, physicians, nurses, psychiatrists, psychologists, priests, and others. Seven years later, survival data for the 224 women were carefully analyzed. Among the patients who had no confidants, the seven-year survival rate was 56.3 percent. Among the women who confided in at least one person, the seven-year survival rate was 66.2 percent. And the survival rate for women reporting two or more confidants was increased even further, to 76 percent.

As the authors acknowledged, the results of this study achieved only borderline statistical significance and must be interpreted with caution.

Nonetheless, no other variables among the women were identified to account for the differences in their survival.

It is important to mention that other well-designed studies have been published that did *not* show any survival advantage among cancer patients who participated in a variety of support groups or other psychosocial interventions. This is not surprising. At the very least, however, the results of all these studies remain intriguing, and they emphasize the need and value of further research in this area.

There are many things you can do as a cancer patient to access the benefits of psychosocial support. As you get started, the following points are helpful to bear in mind:

1. **SEEK OUT MULTIPLE SOURCES OF SUPPORT.** One of the most interesting findings of the Maunsell study was that improvement in survival did not seem to be related to the *type* of confidant the women reported talking to. Whether the confidant was a family member, friend, clergy, nurse, doctor, or other type of confidant, the important element was the trust the patient was able to place in another human being.

For the great majority of cancer patients, family is the foundation of the emotional support system, and there is absolutely no question that strong family ties are tremendously beneficial in the journey through cancer. But cancer patients must realize their families can't "do it all." The intimacy and intensity of family relationships can be a great source of strength. However, the very nature of family ties can also inhibit patients from sharing difficult emotions like anger, fear, and despair. Sometimes it is much easier, and more helpful, to share troubling feelings like these with more neutral listeners.

In a similar way, family members of cancer patients should not feel compelled to take on sole responsibility for their loved one's emotional well-being. Whether acknowledged or not, family members of cancer patients are often under great stress themselves. Support can often be as important, and vital, for them as for the patient.

2. **ONCE YOUR SUPPORT NETWORK IS IN PLACE, USE IT TO THE FULLEST.** Confide in your confidants. Allow yourself to feel

whatever you are feeling, even if it is weak, scared, or angry. Acknowledge the fact that you need help.

Even patients who seem stoically self-sufficient at the outset of treatment often come to realize their need for support. To the extent that they have denied this very human need, they can set themselves up for sudden and unexpected overflows of emotion that may be overwhelming. Cancer demands that you recognize the full range of your feelings, that you share them in appropriate settings, and that you use them to make yourself stronger and healthier. This is an opportunity to experience a kind of trust and growth that many people have never allowed themselves to experience before in their lives. It is also an opportunity to allow those who love and care about you to be able to show and give their love. As difficult as it may seem at first, allow yourself to take full advantage of the support that others want to offer you at this critical time.

3. EVEN IF YOU CHOOSE TO HIDE YOUR ILLNESS, DON'T HIDE IT FROM YOURSELF. Although great progress has been made in controlling the side effects of cancer treatment, many of them still remain. Hair loss still occurs with a number of chemotherapy drugs. Radiation may redden or burn the skin. Some patients may also experience nausea, fatigue, or weight loss during treatment. How to deal with these side effects is a personal matter. The choice of whom to tell about the illness is also a highly individual decision, even if there are no visible signs of the disease.

Whatever approach you take, it's important to be totally honest with yourself about what you are experiencing. Despite the obvious courage of cancer patients, some feel a real sense of shame about their disease. A kind of hiding instinct may appear, which can undermine emotional well-being and complicate the experience of treatment. It is important that you resist this instinct if it is causing you to feel isolated or limited in your options.

You may choose to wear wigs, scarves, baseball hats, or makeup—or you may want the world to see you exactly as you are. This is one time in life in which any choice can be the right one, as long as it comes from self-acceptance and a desire for self-expression.

4. COMMUNICATE WITH PRESENT AND FORMER CANCER PATIENTS. Ultimately, no one—not family members, nor friends, nor physicians—can know how the journey through cancer *feels* from a patient's perspective, unless they have been through it themselves. Oncologists may have administered chemotherapy to thousands of people, yet after only one treatment a patient will know more about the experience than the doctor. That is why it is so important to make contact with people who have firsthand knowledge of what you are going through.

The best way to overcome a sense of isolation is to realize you really *are not* isolated. Many, many people have been exactly where you are now and survived. Many others state unequivocally that their lives were undeniably transformed *for the better* by their experience with cancer. Cancer patients have so much to share with one another that can be found nowhere else. Despite the seriousness of this illness, there is no question that it can be an extraordinary opportunity to give and receive advice, wisdom, and love. The support of others who have "been there" can be vitally important in helping you seize and make the most of these opportunities.

FINDING THE SUPPORT THAT'S RIGHT FOR YOU

Today hundreds of psychosocial resources are available to cancer patients. Some, like talking to a clergy member or other spiritual advisor, have existed for as long as human beings have experienced illness. Others, like support groups and other psychosocial and educational programs, have been around for years and are becoming more available and sophisticated every day. A list of helpful cancer support organizations is provided in Appendix 2, and I strongly urge patients and family members to take advantage of them.

Still others are quite new, such as on-line chat groups or message boards. I personally believe that the Internet provides astonishing opportunities for many patients and their families. A few clicks of the mouse can bring you up-to-the-minute, firsthand information about your diagnosis. It can also put you directly in contact with patients, physicians, publications, and leading cancer centers around the country, if not the world. In terms of psychosocial support, you can instantly interact in real time with people who are exactly where you are right now in the journey through cancer—and it's a lot easier to go on a rafting trip with other travelers than to take off in a rowboat all by yourself. A list of valuable Internet resources is provided in Appendix 3.

One of the Internet's advantages is the anonymity of the participants, since there are many instances in which communication is easier if no one knows who you are. However, the Internet is no substitute for human contact.

Support groups may at times seem more challenging, but they offer something that can only come from sitting down and spending time with other human beings. How this works is a mystery, but it is true. The experience of human beings gathering together to offer each other love and support has existed for millennia. The benefits of that experience are clear and profound.

It is also no exaggeration to say that support group participation can sometimes make the critical difference between patients giving up or fighting for their lives. It can also save a spouse or caregiver from becoming completely overwhelmed by the experience of their loved one's illness. This aspect of the healing process is so important that I'm confident it will soon become a standard component of medical care throughout the United States and elsewhere.

In view of all the evidence regarding the benefits of psychosocial support programs, why do a surprising number of patients still resist participating in them or in other forms of counseling? I believe there are several answers to this, and it is valuable to look closely at each of them. If you are a cancer patient, or if someone close to you has cancer, ask yourself whether you recognize any of these feelings:

• *Do you feel uncomfortable attending a support group because you're "just not someone who joins groups"?* Many people value autonomy and independence as an important aspect of character. They simply aren't at ease with "joining"—whether it's a political movement, a charitable organization, or a support group. Cancer, however, is something entirely new in a patient's life, and everyone can benefit from new ways of helping to deal with the illness. This is not a matter of forsaking basic identity. It is simply an opportunity to introduce some flexibility into a situation where flexibility can be of real benefit.

• *Do you feel that psychosocial support would violate your identity as someone who doesn't need help?* When cancer strikes, your sense of self-sufficiency can receive a sudden and shocking blow. This causes some patients to retreat from others just at the moment when others are needed. What is really called for is a recognition that *you do need support.* No matter how strong you are, or how highly you value your independence, trying to go through cancer alone is a mistake. Often it is simply the fear of admitting this that causes patients or family members to avoid support groups or other forms of psychosocial support.

• *Do you envision a support group as a threatening, unsafe, or depressing environment?* When a cancer patient wants to stay away from other cancer patients, this might really be an attempt to get away from himself or herself. It is often a way of unconsciously saying cancer is still "the enemy"—and that being close to people with cancer might lead to a deeply unsettling recognition of "the enemy within me." This often consumes significantly more precious time and energy than patients appreciate. A much more effective approach is to accurately identify what or who the real enemy is. Or, even better, to abandon the notion that there is an enemy at all.

• *If you were to take part in a support group, do you fear exploring emotions that might come to the surface?* A typical response to cancer is to try to shore up our areas of weakness, because cancer is going to require all the strength and attention we can muster. However, it takes a lot of energy to keep angers, fears, pains, resentments, and frustrations bottled up. Acknowledging them and working through them can be intimidating. Nevertheless, doing so is extremely important and worthwhile—and, as we have seen, may be life-saving as well. This is especially true since unexplored feelings can intensify under the stress of illness and may express themselves in ways that are hurtful, not only to patients but also to those close to them.

• *Would a support group violate your rules about sharing your feelings with strangers?* If all the world is indeed a stage, cancer pushes patients right onto the center of it and challenges them to start reciting their best lines.

Many patients, however, would rather remain in the wings. It is only in the past few decades that the idea of expressing thoughts and feelings has begun to gain acceptance in our culture. For the generation of the Depression and World War Two, what is now called denial was known as toughness and the ability to keep your mouth shut. But those qualities, even if cultivated over a lifetime, come at a price that a cancer patient can hardly afford. The notion that sharing your feelings somehow diminishes your strength is, simply, wrong. In fact, the opposite is true.

• *Would attending a support group make it more difficult for you to deny you have cancer?* Some patients try to deal with their illness "as if nothing has happened." These are people who rush from the hospital or from a chemotherapy treatment directly back to their well-established routine, whether it be golf, gin rummy, or trading commodities futures. Of course, this is every patient's right—but it is also a missed opportunity. Tremendous insight and growth can be gained at this time, but the opportunity is lost when you run headlong away from your immediate experience back to the known and familiar. Cancer must be seen for what it is. It is much more than an annoyance or an inconvenience in your daily routine—no matter how much patients may at times wish to deny this. The risk of wearing blinders in cancer is that they can suddenly come off. Without becoming obsessed with cancer, therefore, it is important for patients to give the illness its proper place and significance in their lives.

TYPES OF SUPPORT GROUPS

Just as chemotherapy, radiation, and surgery have evolved to focus much more precisely on the needs of individual patients, psychosocial support programs are evolving as well.

Cancer patients often respond quite differently to various kinds of psychosocial interventions. Some patients respond more readily to individual counseling while others prefer group discussion. It is important for everyone involved to accurately define their needs and to choose the kind of support that serves them best.

Patricia Fobair, a clinical social worker at Stanford University, has described a variety of group settings that are often employed for cancer patients, family members, and caregivers. Among the most widely used group formats are the following:

• **Open-ended groups** are probably the most common setting for psychosocial support in cancer. These groups may include any combination of patients, family members, friends, and caregivers, or they may be limited to only one category. Typically, groups meet on a regular basis with social workers, clinicians, or even former patients acting as facilitators. Often a group will continue meeting for several years. Many patients prefer this continuity rather than a shorter-term arrangement. Although patients may initially feel apprehensive about joining a support group, the vast majority find the experience beneficial in terms of their ability to deal with fear and anxiety, to communicate their feelings and concerns, and to gain vitally helpful emotional support at critical times.

• **Patient education groups** focus on the clinical and practical issues of cancer. For some patients, mastering the facts of their illness and its treatment can provide therapeutic benefit even if emotional issues are never directly addressed. This may be especially true for patients with an intellectual orientation to life. One of the most difficult aspects of cancer can be the impression that your life is being taken over by something confusing and beyond comprehension. When psychosocial support is used to dispel that notion, a major obstacle is removed.

• **Cognitive-behavioral groups** teach coping techniques of mindful awareness and positive reinforcement. For example, patients may learn valuable ways to stop themselves from slipping into depressive thought patterns or to replace negative thoughts with a positive or uplifting affirmation. Even learning to monitor and be aware of thoughts that occur during the day can be very helpful.

• **Supportive-expressive groups** encourage shared feelings and empathy among members not only during formal group sessions but outside the meetings as well. This aspect of psychosocial support has also been effective in areas outside cancer care. Twelve-step programs, for example, have different goals and intentions than cancer support groups, but they also encourage members to become part of one another's lives outside the formal meeting. The power of this approach cannot be denied.

Once again, as we gain greater understanding of how psychosocial interventions can impact the lives of cancer patients and their family members in profound ways, a high level of psychosocial support will become a requirement for any oncologist's office or certified cancer center. If a cancer patient is having bone pain or mouth sores associated with chemotherapy, it is the physician's responsibility to provide a medication that brings relief. Similarly, when a patient is suffering from isolation, loneliness, or others forms of emotional distress, and especially when we know how this can adversely impact his or her experience, I believe we have a responsibility to address this aspect of the patient's needs. This is not "window dressing" on cancer treatment. It is an absolutely essential component.

6

LEVEL THREE:
THE BODY AS GARDEN

THE NATURAL HEALING FORCE WITHIN EACH OF
US IS THE GREATEST FORCE IN GETTING WELL.

—HIPPOCRATES

Years ago, when I first began to explore the great spiritual and healing traditions of the East, my travels took me to India, Nepal, China, and Tibet. One metaphor from the traditions of those countries captured my attention—the human body seen as a garden, and the physician as someone who tends it. I was particularly impressed by the contrast of these images with those from the West, in which the human body is often regarded as a machine and the physician as a mechanic. I fell in love with the image of "the body as garden," and it still inspires me. It also serves as the inspiration for Level Three of this program.

For both patients and doctors, the idea of the body as garden opens up new ways of thinking about ourselves—and about medicine and healing as well. It opens up tremendous opportunities for us all to play genuinely positive roles in the healing process. It gives each of us a chance to ask, "What can I do to cultivate the garden of my being in such a way that the fruits and flowers of health, well-being, and self-knowledge can blossom and grow? What can I do to fertilize and till the soil of my being in order to accomplish this?"

Within each of us are deep and powerful mechanisms of healing that can make an enormous difference in getting well. One of your most important objectives as a cancer patient should be to cleanse and nourish your body in a way that allows those inner healing mechanisms to flourish as fully as possible.

When a garden is carefully tended, destructive life-forms like weeds or parasites may still appear, but they are much less likely to take over. They can be dealt with while they are still in an easily manageable form. Making a garden healthy also requires giving it adequate nutrients and water, and turning the soil so the earth mixes with fresh air. Removing toxins and other harmful substances from the environment is essential, along with making sure that the garden has plenty of sunlight. By tending to all these things, a gardener gives nature the fullest possible opportunity to come into congruence with his or her wishes.

If a garden is neglected, another side of nature is likely to assert itself. Weeds are just as "natural" as roses, but they're out of synch with our ultimate interests. They're also out of synch with all the other plants in the garden. They can quickly usurp the space and nourishment of the other plants, often killing them in the process. The weeds can also eventually choke off one another and cause their own death.

This is as close to a perfect analogy with cancer as we are likely to find. Good nutrition, exercise, and a life that is emotionally and spiritually fulfilled is not a guarantee that cancer will be prevented, let alone cured. However, actively pursuing all these can help—sometimes very significantly.

Level Three of this program is an invitation to develop an entirely new, ongoing relationship with your body. This new relationship begins by seeing your body as a garden that needs nurturing and care, as well as sufficient space and sunshine in which to heal and grow. Your body is not a machine that was created simply to carry out the will of its owner. The idea that the body must do the bidding of the human ego rarely works in the journey through cancer—in fact, it can be counterproductive. Your body is a living, breathing organism, a focal point of energy, information, intelligence, and growth. And healing from cancer is, ultimately, an organic process that requires many ingredients. An element of mystery also accompanies this process. Consciously connecting with that mystery can be healing in and of itself.

But a new perspective is not all that is required for a successful journey through cancer. On a very practical level, a wide variety of viewpoints, philosophies, and treatments for cancer are now available. These compete for attention, and sometimes are even openly in conflict. For every patient, they also raise complex but vitally important questions:

- How can I gain maximum benefit from conventional cancer treatment, while minimizing risk and discomfort?
- What are the proper roles for complementary and alternative therapies in my cancer treatment?
- Is there anything I should be eating during my treatment, and what should I not eat?
- What vitamins, minerals, and supplements should I take?
- Should I be taking antioxidants, and if so, what kinds?
- How much should I exercise, or should I just rest as much as possible?
- Is it okay for me to have a massage if I have cancer?
- What can I do to minimize the side effects of my cancer treatment?
- How can I talk to my doctor about my interest in complementary and alternative medicine?
- What about the Eastern healing traditions? Do they have anything to offer me?

This chapter sorts out the enormous confusion that patients and family members so often encounter in dealing with these questions. It provides a framework within which different approaches can find an appropriate place without overwhelming one another, and without interfering with the most important clinical aspects of a patient's care.

While I strongly believe that conventional therapies are the foundation of effective cancer treatment, I also believe there are important roles for many of the other approaches that are available.

Let's define some of the terms in greater detail:

- **Complementary medicine** refers to the wide variety of physical, mental, emotional, and spiritual techniques that can benefit patients at all points in the journey through cancer. These include diet and nutritional programs, herbs, supplements, aromatherapy, massage, exercise, yoga, relaxation, journaling, visualization and guided imagery, acupuncture, chiropractic, homeopathy, Therapeutic Touch, Reiki therapy, and much more. In general, these may be used along with conventional treatment, hence the term *complementary*.

• **Alternative medicine** encompasses methods that are sometimes used by cancer patients instead of conventional cancer treatment. A defining characteristic of these methods is that they are scientifically *unproven* to be of benefit as a treatment of cancer. Some are even potentially dangerous. If they are used at all, and particularly as primary therapy for cancer, I believe it should be with great caution, and only when there are no proven therapies available that can be of benefit.

Alternative treatments include Burzinski antineoplastons; the Hoxsey Method; the Contreras Method; DMSO; Kelly metabolic therapy; live cell therapy; the Gerson Method; the Greek Cancer Cure (Alivizatos therapy); high-dose intravenous vitamins; shark cartilage; Essiac tea; hydrazine sulfate; CanCell (Entelev); hyperoxygenation therapies; immunoaugmentative therapies; Iscador (mistletoe extract); Laetrile (amygdalin); Livingston-Wheeler therapy; macrobiotic diets; "psychic surgery"; and the Revici Method, among others.

• **Eastern healing traditions** refer to the ancient healing methods of India *(Ayurveda)*, China *(Traditional Chinese Medicine)*, and Tibet *(Tibetan Medicine)*, among others. Elements of all these traditions can be used in either complementary *or* alternative ways, depending upon the circumstances and the intentions of patients and practitioners.

A working knowledge of these ideas and principles can be very helpful to cancer patients and their families. We'll now look at them more closely.

COMPLEMENTARY MEDICINE

Diet and Nutrition

In our image of the body as garden, diet and nutrition correspond to fertilization of the soil. The importance of this is fairly self-evident. "You are what you eat" is a phrase that is well known, and on a basic level our physical selves are indeed an expression of the material we take in. If we are ill, quite often, although by no means always, this may be in some way related to what we have eaten. Furthermore, by eating and drinking with greater knowledge and care, perhaps additional illness can be prevented.

The question of how this applies to cancer is one that scientists have been asking for a long time, and although some answers have finally emerged many areas of confusion and uncertainty remain. As a first step toward eliminating this confusion, it is helpful to recognize that diet and nutrition play different roles at three distinct phases in a cancer patient's life: prior to diagnosis, during treatment, and after treatment has been completed.

Let's look at each of these areas separately.

1. The role of diet and nutrition in the prevention or causation of cancer

Cancer has plagued human beings for thousands of years, and the disease is found in populations with a wide variety of dietary habits and customs. It is now quite clear, however, based upon hundreds of studies in the medical literature, that diet and nutrition do indeed play a significant role in cancer. The American Cancer Society estimates that diet is a primary factor in a third of cancer deaths. But the precise nature of diet's role has yet to be defined.

Several things contribute to this lack of clarity. Primary among them is the great diversity found among different cancers and the individuals in which they arise. Not only does everyone eat different foods at different times of the day, but the foods are prepared differently, combined differently, and metabolized differently by different individuals. Research on diet and nutrition is also costly, time-consuming, and logistically challenging. Nonetheless, it is possible to make some general statements about the role of nutrition in the prevention of cancer, or in contributing to its cause:

A PLANT-BASED DIET IS PROTECTIVE AGAINST SOME CANCERS. The vast majority of studies regarding diet and cancer published in the medical literature suggest a significant protective effect of diets rich in fruits and vegetables. These contain substances known as *phytonutrients* (from the Greek word *phyto,* meaning plant), which are believed to protect against cancer by a number of different mechanisms.

One of those mechanisms involves highly active molecules known as *free radicals,* which are present in every cell of the body. These can damage cellular DNA and other molecules in ways that initiate tumor development. Fruits and vegetables are key sources of *antioxidants,* which play an important role in preventing the damage to cells caused by these free radicals.

Some of the best-known antioxidants are vitamins C, E, and *beta carotene,* which are found in a wide variety of fruits and vegetables. *Lycopene* is another well-known antioxidant; it gives tomatoes their red color. Other examples include *polyphenols,* which occur in green tea, and *glutathione,* which is found in fruits and vegetables and is also created in the body from amino acids.

Numerous research studies indicate that people who consume foods rich in antioxidants have a lower risk of developing certain types of cancer. It is important to note, however, that commercially prepared antioxidant supplements have not consistently been shown to provide similar statistical benefits. In fact, beta carotene supplements were shown in one study to *increase* the risk of lung cancer among subjects who smoke. Despite the lack of scientifically proven benefit, consumption of antioxidant supplements on a regular basis has become one of the fastest-growing health-related industries in the United States.

Green leafy vegetables such as broccoli, cabbage, Brussels sprouts, and cauliflower (called *cruciferous* vegetables) are rich in other phytonutrients, notably *indoles* and *sulphoraphane.* These are believed to protect against cancer by mechanisms that are different than those of antioxidants, including removing estrogen and other potentially harmful substances from cells.

Resveratrol, which is present in red grapes and red wine, is yet another phytonutrient that is believed to protect against cancer by inhibiting enzymes involved in inflammation.

Soy products, including tofu, miso, and soy milk contain chemicals called *isoflavones,* which act as weak estrogens and are believed to help reduce the risk of hormone-related cancers. Studies have shown that women who eat soy products such as tofu and soy milk have a lower incidence of breast cancer. This may be part of the reason why Asian women are at lower risk for developing this disease.

Garlic contains chemicals called *allyl sulfides*, which are believed to lower cancer risk by influencing the metabolism of cancer-causing substances in the liver. Studies have suggested that people with diets high in garlic may have a lower risk of stomach cancer.

A word should be mentioned about *selenium*, another well-known antioxidant that is found in vegetables, as well as in fish, meats, and nuts. A 1996 study suggested that individuals who consumed a daily 200 mcg selenium supplement for an average of 4.5 years had significantly lower incidence and mortality from lung, colorectal, and prostate cancers. These intriguing results suggest that regular consumption of antioxidant supplements may indeed prove beneficial in helping reduce the risk of developing cancer. Further studies are underway.

HIGH DIETARY CONSUMPTION OF FAT CONTRIBUTES TO THE DEVELOPMENT OF SOME CANCERS. Although the role of fat in the promotion of cancer is still under investigation, there is important evidence of its involvement. Much of the evidence comes from epidemiologic studies that indicate that a "Western" high-fat diet is associated with increased risk of hormone-related cancers (such as breast, endometrium, and prostate) and gastrointestinal cancers (such as colon, rectum, and gallbladder). It is not clear whether the associations are directly causal or whether they are confounded by numerous other possible factors. Some of the potentially complicating factors include total caloric intake, overall body weight, exercise habits, possible contamination by pesticides and hormones, dietary fiber content, and cooking methods.

It is also not clear if the observed associations of fat consumption and cancer risk relate to specific types of fat (such as saturated, unsaturated, or polyunsaturated). Some research suggests that saturated fats (found in meat and dairy products) and omega-6 polyunsaturated fatty acids (found in corn and safflower oils) may be more closely linked with cancer risk than other types of fat. Other research suggests that omega-3 polyunsaturated fatty acids (found in flaxseed and cold-water fish) may be protective against cancer as well as heart disease. Olive oil, which contains a monounsaturated fat called oleic acid, has also been suggested to have a protective effect against some cancers.

Despite the unresolved controversies regarding the precise role of fat and cancer risk, numerous organizations, including the National Research Council, the National Academy of Sciences, and the American Cancer Society, among others, have recommended reducing fat intake to 30 percent or less of total calories. They have also recommended increasing dietary consumption of fruits and vegetables and reducing alcohol consumption.

ALCOHOL CONSUMPTION CONTRIBUTES TO CANCER RISK. The link between smoking and cancer has now been so well established that it hardly needs to be repeated here. Although the link between alcohol and cancer has not received the attention that has been focused on smoking, it is also very well established. Drinking seems to amplify the effects of carcinogens, particularly tobacco smoke. It also causes irritation to tissues of the mouth, esophagus, larynx, stomach, and liver in ways that might contribute to the development of cancer in these organs. By other mechanisms, it also increases the risk of breast cancer.

But perhaps the most significant effect of alcohol consumption is the fact that it tends to promote unhealthy eating and lifestyle habits in general. When people are drinking, they're usually not eating broccoli and carrots along with their cocktails. Individuals who drink heavily develop cancer at a rate *ten times higher* than the overall population.

Having made these general statements, it should be emphasized once again that the precise role of diet and nutrition in cancer still remains controversial. As often happens in science, two articles of faith about the relationship between diet and cancer have recently been called into question.

Since the late 1960s, it was believed that a high-fiber diet helped to prevent colon cancer. In January of 1999, however, results from a twenty-five-year study involving more than 88,000 women showed that those who consumed the most fiber—up to 25 grams per day—contracted colon cancer with *virtually the same frequency* as women whose daily fiber intake was only 10 grams or less. Aside from what this study says about fiber and cancer prevention, it reveals the tenuous nature of even the most "certain" information about this disease. Although a reasonable amount of fiber remains an important component of a healthy diet, this lesson should be kept in mind by everyone who is concerned about cancer and its causes.

Similarly, the idea that a low-fat diet would lower the risk of breast cancer was widely accepted over many years, popularized in numerous magazine articles and several books. In March 1999, a study involving 2,956 women reported finding *no evidence* that lower intake of fat or specific major types of fat was associated with a decreased risk of breast cancer.

We want to believe we can avoid cancer by eating healthy foods, and indeed a good diet can make the difference for a sizable number of people. While I certainly advise people to eat plenty of fruits and vegetables—and even to consider daily vitamin, mineral, and antioxidant supplements—I do not believe this should be done simply in order to avoid cancer. Throughout this book we are making the point that *no decisions should be made from fear,* whether it is eating broccoli or taking chemotherapy.

In my opinion, the best reason to follow the principles of a healthy diet—and a healthy lifestyle in general—is because doing so will yield significant benefits in *every area of your life.* Along with greater energy, improved physical health, increased vitality, and an enhanced sense of well-being, you will have greater awareness, increased clarity of mind, and expanded opportunities to achieve your life's deeper goals.

2. The role of diet and nutrition during cancer treatment

The role of diet and nutrition in the treatment of cancer has been hotly debated in recent years, particularly among patients who want to do everything possible to help themselves get well. Unfortunately, despite good intentions, this subject can become an area of great pain and confusion for patients and family members.

Adequate nutrition is an important concern for everyone. Quite often, it is even *more important* for people with cancer. But in many instances, nutritional concerns are not as important—particularly in the short term—as they might appear to the individuals involved, or as sometimes suggested by alternative practitioners. The urgency and fear felt by patients and their loved ones around issues of diet and nutrition is often magnified, burdensome, and unnecessary.

Balance and perspective are the key elements needed here. Nutrition is rarely a "make-or-break" issue for people in cancer treatment. In the majority of cases, nutrition has a *relative* importance that must be factored into a long list of other priorities and concerns. It should be given *appropriate* attention—not too little, but not too much either. Furthermore, appropriate attention differs among patients, the various stages of their illness, and the treatment they will be receiving.

Many patients have early-stage cancers that need only limited, defined periods of adjuvant treatment. For them, the short-term issue of what to eat during their care is usually much less important than what they eat during the rest of their lives after their treatment is completed. On the other hand, if a patient has metastatic cancer and will require chemotherapy or radiation over an extended period of time, issues of nutritional support become much more important.

There is no question that during all phases of cancer treatment the body needs adequate vitamins, minerals, and calories. For many patients this will not be a problem, but for others maintaining adequate nutrition is more easily said than done.

Several forms of cancer are associated with loss of appetite and a diminished sense of taste. Cancer treatments themselves can also produce these effects. Nausea and mouth sores sometimes associated with chemotherapy do not inspire patients to eat big, healthy meals. Another common problem, called *esophagitis,* can occur in patients receiving radiation therapy for lung cancer, esophageal cancer, or lymphomas in the chest. This condition is a radiation-induced "sunburn" of the inner lining of the esophagus, and it can make swallowing food or even liquids extremely difficult or painful. Patients undergoing radiation treatments for cancers of the mouth, throat, or neck can have similar problems.

General Diet and Nutrition Guidelines During Cancer Treatment

With the above as a preamble, here are some simple guidelines that can be helpful to patients. They can be useful for spouses and family members as well.

- Adopt a more plant-based diet.
- Try to eat several servings of fruits and vegetables each day.
- Cut back on your consumption of red meat. You can replenish your intake of protein by eating beans, fish, lentils, or nuts.
- Start eating whole grains every day, including brown rice, lentils, and buckwheat.
- Buy a juicer, and start drinking fresh fruit and vegetable juices daily.
- Avoid fried, greasy, or fatty foods.
- Minimize your intake of refined sugar.
- Minimize your intake of alcohol.
- Keep yourself well hydrated. Drink at least 6–8 glasses of spring water each day.
- Consider supplementing your diet with a high-quality multivitamin once or twice a day. If you have difficulty swallowing pills, try vitamin powders that you can mix in fruit juices or water.
- Consider other nutritional supplements, including liquid trace minerals and protein drinks.
- Above all, avoid making your diet another source of stress. Don't feel guilty about eating foods you like, and don't feel obligated to eat foods or diets you don't want.

Despite anecdotal accounts of the benefits of intensive nutritional programs, including high-dose intravenous vitamin regimens, cleansing diets, and macrobiotics, none of these approaches has been scientifically proven to be helpful. Sometimes they also pose real risks and potential adverse effects.

This is particularly true of antioxidants when taken concurrently with conventional cancer treatment. Studies have suggested that patients who take antioxidant supplements during chemotherapy or radiation may experience fewer side effects. This occurs presumably because of the antioxidants' ability to reduce the toxic effects of the treatment on normal cells and tissues. Unfortunately, the antioxidants may be simultaneously reducing the effects of the treatment on the *cancer cells*. Patients may think the antioxidants are helping them, when in fact they may be causing harm. The answer is not yet known. For this reason, I generally advise patients to avoid taking antioxidants until their chemotherapy or radiation treatments are completed.

Remember, everyone is unique, and your needs may vary at different times during your treatment. If you have any questions about your diet, and especially about the appropriateness of taking vitamins, minerals, antioxidants, or other nutritional supplements, it is important to consult your oncologist.

Some Advice for Family Members

It is very difficult to see a loved one in the midst of a serious illness. Quite naturally everyone feels an instinctive desire to help. Suggestions about diet and nutrition are often the vehicles people choose for expressing their love and concern. Family or friends may recommend macrobiotic diets, teas, liquid herbal extracts, vitamins, pills, and other dietary options. But well-meaning people do not always understand the real needs of patients during treatment. And patients themselves may not be able to express their needs as clearly or as forcefully as they might wish.

Beyond helping the patient get the best possible medical care, perhaps the most important task for family members is to *accept and support your loved one's choices.* Consciously choosing to honor and respect a patient's decisions is one of the greatest gifts you can give. This comes up frequently in the area of nutrition, where family members and friends often feel compelled to offer food or dietary suggestions, even when patients are clearly not interested.

Paul Delaney is a seventy-four-year-old man undergoing combined radiation and chemotherapy treatment for esophageal cancer. He is a robust, jolly person who always loved to eat, and his wife loved to cook for him. He had hardly been sick in his entire life until several months ago, when he began to notice food getting stuck in his throat. Medical evaluation revealed a tumor obstructing a good portion of his esophagus.

During the first month of his treatment, Mr. Delaney did extremely well. He had no nausea or vomiting, kept active every day, and started swallowing food more easily soon after his treatment began. His appetite was good, and he even started gaining weight. Following his second cycle of chemotherapy, he began to feel run-down and tired. His appetite began to diminish, and he started to feel a burning sensation in his esophagus from the radiation. He started eating less.

Careful medical evaluation of his condition showed no other worri-some findings or cause for alarm. His weight loss was minimal. I informed Mr. Delaney and his wife that his symptoms were entirely in line with what one might expect in a man his age at this point in treatment and offered him appropriate medications to alleviate his symptoms.

Mr. Delaney, reassured, was confident about going ahead with his remaining treatments. But for Mrs. Delaney, a big problem had arisen.

"Doctor, what am I going to do?" she said with exasperation. "My husband won't eat! I try to feed him ten times a day, but he refuses every-thing. It's driving me crazy! You have to do something. If *you* tell him to eat, then he will listen. But he won't listen to me."

I asked Mr. Delaney if this was true.

"Well," he replied, "I just don't feel like eating too much right now. I'm tired, and I don't have much of an appetite. I don't want to eat any big meals, but she keeps on pushing me to eat more."

"You *have* to eat more, Paul," Mrs. Delaney interrupted. "You're eat-ing like a bird, and you're going to waste away and starve to death if you don't eat more."

"See? She won't let up on me," Mr. Delaney said. "I tell her to leave me alone, but she won't stop. All day long, it's *eat, eat, eat*. But I don't *want* to eat. What should I do?"

This is a scenario that oncologists encounter virtually every day. Responding most effectively to it requires insight into all dimensions of what is *really* going on.

I responded to Mr. Delaney's question by once again examining him carefully and reviewing his chart, and I then gently reassured Mrs. Delaney that her husband's medical tests had revealed no other cause for alarm. He had lost only three pounds over the prior few weeks, and I reassured her that this small amount of weight loss was not dangerous. He was by no means at risk of "starving to death." Fifty years of her home cooking had boosted Paul's weight to over two hundred pounds.

Then I turned to Paul, and said, "Mr. Delaney, may I ask you a question?"

"Sure," he said.

"Why do you think Mrs. Delaney keeps trying to get you to eat so much?"

Mr. Delaney paused for a long time, and then he started to choke up. He was a proud man, and he almost never allowed himself to cry. Fighting back tears, he said, "I don't know."

"No, really, Paul. Why do you think Mrs. Delaney wants you to eat so much?"

After another long pause, he finally said, "Well, I guess she does it because she loves me."

"I think that's very true, Paul," I said. "And why else does she try to get you to eat so much?"

"Well," he said, after another long pause, "I guess she does it because she doesn't want me to be sick."

I looked at Mrs. Delaney and asked, "Is that true?"

She nodded her head in agreement.

I looked back at Mr. Delaney, and asked, "And why doesn't she want you to be sick?"

Mr. Delaney now paused for a very long time, before answering softly, "I guess because she doesn't want me to die."

I then asked Paul to look at his wife. Her eyes were filled with tears, and she reached out and hugged him. "That's right, Paul," she said. "I love you so much, and I'm afraid to lose you. I want you to eat so you'll be healthy. I don't want to lose you."

This was a beautiful breakthrough in their journey together. It was also a moment of truth and a turning point of sorts.

"May I offer you a suggestion?" I asked.

"Yes, please," they both replied.

"Okay," I said. "First of all, I want to acknowledge you both for telling the truth the way you just have. It is so beautiful and moving for me to see this. Thank you.

"Now, Mr. Delaney," I continued, "do you realize that asking Mrs. Delaney to stop offering you food would be very difficult and painful for her?"

"Yes," he replied. "I can see that."

"And, Mrs. Delaney, can you see how your continuous insistence that Paul eat all the time, and that he eat bigger meals than he really wants, is only causing him pain and making him feel *worse* than he already does?"

"Yes," she said, with an obviously heavy heart. "I can see that now. I didn't see it before."

"I'm sure you didn't," I said, "because I know you only want to help your husband."

"Oh yes," she said. "That's true."

"Great," I continued. "My recommendation is that you have an agreement with each other that looks something like this." I turned to Mr. Delaney. "What I'd like to suggest is that you agree to allow Mrs. Delaney to offer you food, but no more than *three times a day*. Will that work for you?"

"Sure," Mr. Delaney replied.

"And will you also agree that if you feel hungry, or if you want to eat something special, that you will ask Mrs. Delaney to make it for you?"

"Why, sure," he said. "That's easy."

"Terrific. I can feel we're making progress here."

I then turned to Mrs. Delaney, and said, "Now, Mrs. Delaney, if Paul says, 'No thank you, honey. I don't want to eat right now,' are you willing to agree that you will ask him 'Are you sure?' *only one time*? Can you agree to that?"

"Well, I guess so," she replied cautiously. "But what if he doesn't eat at all? What am I supposed to do then?"

"If that happens I want you to call me, and let me know about it. If I'm not here, speak to any other of the staff members, and they will let me know right away. I don't want you to be worrying yourself sick over this. We will keep a very close watch on Mr. Delaney right along with you, and make sure that he is not losing too much weight. Okay?"

"Okay," she said. "That'll be fine."

Mr. and Mrs. Delaney's experience is a human and understandable occurrence on the journey through cancer. Underlying Mrs. Delaney's pain and anguish with regard to her husband's nutritional status is not only her love for him and her fear of losing him, but also a mistaken belief that she is in some way responsible for whether or not he eats. I believe it is absolutely essential for family members and friends to recognize that they are *not responsible* for what their loved one eats or does not eat. Although this is sometimes hard to accept—and unless a clear agreement exists to the contrary—they are not ultimately responsible for *any* aspect of the patient's care.

Let me explain what I mean by this. Although you may be involved in administering medications, changing bandages, or assisting with other aspects of the patient's care, I believe your most helpful role is to be their confidant, family member, lover perhaps, or friend. If you can fully embrace this idea, you will help yourself—and your loved one—more than you can imagine. My strong recommendation for patients and family members is to make a conscious choice to let the patient's physicians and nurses be responsible for the patient's medical welfare. If you have any concerns or anxieties about what is happening to them, medically or nutritionally, address those concerns directly to your loved one's medical team. Also, it is a very good idea to seek out other avenues of support for yourself, such as individual counseling, contact with friends, or support groups where you can find valuable information, insights, and advice.

Here is a summary of these important ideas:

- The helping intentions of family members need to be openly acknowledged. Family members deserve to be heard, understood, and appreciated.
- Family members must accept their proper role as sources of love and support for the patient—rather than assuming responsibility for the patient's nutritional status or medical care on their own.
- Family members should agree they will offer food to the patient no more than three times a day. If the patient declines, they agree to ask "Are you sure?" *only once.*
- The patient agrees to ask for more or different food when he or she wishes.
- Finally, family members must recognize and agree that the patient is a sovereign being who deserves their *unconditional* love and support. This includes supporting their choices about eating whatever and whenever they choose. Family members must acknowledge that the patient can direct *all* aspects of the journey through cancer as he or

she sees fit—*even in ways that are completely different from what family members might wish or choose for themselves.*

3. The role of diet and nutrition after treatment has been completed

A good cancer recovery diet includes the recommendations for diet and nutrition during cancer treatment listed on page 99. It is not surprising that these recommendations can be helpful for everyone, whether they have had cancer or not.

Certainly, there is much more that an individual could explore to maximize health after cancer treatment beyond the above recommendations. Pursuing optimum health is a lifelong and potentially unlimited process. Neither asceticism nor overindulgence are in the best interests of any cancer patient, or any human being. So, after your treatment is completed, by all means eat fruits and vegetables, take vitamins, and drink plenty of water—but don't be afraid to enjoy other foods also. Enjoy life!

In discussing the areas of complementary medicine that follow, it is best to adopt the same approach we have applied to nutrition. The issue is not, "Which herbs, relaxation techniques, homeopathic remedies, or acupuncture treatments should I take to get rid of my cancer?" The more appropriate questions are: *What can help me feel better? What can improve my digestion, benefit my sleep, and enhance my overall health? What makes sense for me at this time in my life?*

Once again, your intention should be learning to care for the garden of your own unique being—with the help, support, and guidance of your doctor, your family, and your friends—so that the fruits and flowers of health, well-being, and self-knowledge can blossom and grow.

Herbs and Supplements

For millions of Americans, herbs and dietary supplements have become full-fledged alternatives to prescription drugs. In this brief discussion, we will make a distinction between the way herbs and supplements are often understood, and used, by patients. While this distinction may not be precise in all instances, I believe it is most helpful from a practical standpoint:

• Herbs and herbal compounds are usually taken with a specific medicinal intent. They are commonly used to deal with particular clinical problems, which may be chronic or acute and can range from tension headaches to advanced cancer.

For many people, one of the real attractions of herbal medications is that they are "natural" products. They come from trees and plants rather than from laboratories and chemicals. In the minds of many individuals, "natural" generally means good, not dangerous, and nontoxic. Most herbs are indeed safe and free of side effects. But no substance, including water, is without risk in every patient and under all circumstances.

Conventional chemotherapy is often criticized for its toxicity, particularly by adherents of natural forms of healing, but many people are not aware that some important chemotherapy drugs are derived from plants. Nor do many people realize that herbs can be very powerful and should not be used indiscriminately—particularly when undergoing cancer treatment. Herbs have been used for centuries by different cultures around the world for the treatment of cancer, although most herbal cancer remedies are unproven by Western scientific standards. In addition, herbs are sometimes used to ameliorate the side effects of cancer and cancer treatment. Examples include St. John's wort for depression, ginger for nausea, and aloe for topical irritations related to radiation.

The fact that herbs are derived from plants does not mean they are without risks, especially when taken concurrently with chemotherapy or other prescribed medications. Many herbs are metabolized in the liver, where they can interfere with the metabolism of numerous commonly prescribed drugs. One example involves a drug called *coumadin*, a blood thinner used to treat blood clots. Oncologists are sometimes puzzled by the inconsistent effects of coumadin on a patient—until they learn that the patient has been taking one or perhaps several herbal preparations that are interfering with the metabolism of the prescribed medication. If you are taking, or are thinking about taking, herbs of any kind—for any purpose—during your cancer treatment, it is important to notify your physician.

I believe it is best to use herbal medications, as with nutrition and other complementary forms of healing, with the intention of bringing love and care to your physical being—nourishing the body as garden—rather than as a specific treatment for your cancer. Resist the temptation to think of herbs as magic potions or as external sources of a quick cure for your illness. Don't put the responsibility for your health on the contents of any bottle, regardless of whether they are "natural" or not. Instead, use them as a means of supporting the healing intention that is present in your mind and heart. This is as true for chemotherapy as it for herbs.

• While herbal medications are commonly used for specific medicinal purposes, nutritional supplements are usually intended to restore or increase the overall energy reserves of the body.

By this definition, supplements include vitamins, trace minerals, antioxidants, protein powders, and substances such as creatine and DHEA. The purpose of these is usually to strengthen general aspects of the physiology rather than to provide relief from specific symptoms. When taken in moderation, most nutritional supplements are harmless, and many individuals feel they are helpful as well. But on a practical level, it is important to be aware of the biological effects of specific substances, both on a short-term and long-term basis. DHEA, for example, has received attention as an anti-aging supplement, but both men and women should be aware that the body metabolizes DHEA into testosterone and estrogen. This could be problematic for individuals who are at high risk for developing prostate or breast cancer. Similarly, as discussed earlier, the interaction of antioxidants with chemotherapy drugs remains at best unclear, and diminished side effects may come at the price of reduced treatment effectiveness.

As with herbs and other forms of complementary therapy, remember to discuss the use of nutritional supplements with your physician, particularly when you are undergoing cancer treatment.

Aromatherapy

For centuries, many of the world's religious traditions have recognized the importance of scent as a stimulus to higher awareness and awareness of the inner self. Incense is a prominent feature of many Christian, Buddhist, Hindu, and other religious ceremonies. The healing power of different aromas has recently come under scientific investigation as well.

Physiologically, the human sense of smell is characterized by a direct connection between the organs of olfactory perception in the nose and the brain's hypothalamus, which regulates functions such as body temperature and growth as well as emotional responses. Aromatherapy uses particular scents to help promote awareness and inner healing responses. Using aromas during cancer treatment is an excellent way to nurture body, mind, heart, and spirit. There are many varieties of scented oils and incense from which to choose. Sandalwood, lavender, and patchouly are especially useful to foster relaxation and a sense of inner peace.

Massage

I have repeatedly been amazed by the benefits of massage for cancer patients. Well-documented physiological effects of massage include pain relief through the release of *endorphins*—the body's natural painkillers—into the bloodstream; heightened immune function; and improved blood flow to vital organs. But the emotional benefits of massage may be even more significant.

For many patients, the loving, conscious touch of a skilled massage therapist just before a chemotherapy treatment can transform the experience from something to be endured into a time they actually look forward to with serenity and gratitude. For loved ones and caregivers, massage can provide an equally important source of respite and rejuvenation.

When massage is administered by a professional therapist, it provides an important source of human contact outside the circle of family and friends. This is valuable not only for patients but also for their loved ones, who often feel that they alone must fulfill all of the patient's needs, often neglecting their own. Massage is an opportunity for tapping into a sense of total receptivity to loving attention from the environment. Anxiety and apprehension are replaced by openness and tranquility, and this fosters healing at every level, for everyone involved.

At one time patients shied away from massage out of fear that it might promote dissemination of cancer cells in the body. For the great majority of cancers this is a myth, but you should consult your doctor before beginning massage therapy. Common sense is also important. Do not massage known points of disease or inflamed areas of the body. Otherwise, there is usually no reason why you cannot enjoy this important, powerful, and enjoyable form of healing.

A number of different styles of massage can be explored by cancer patients and family members. These include the Western styles, which derive from Swedish massage and are usually performed with warmed oils; shiatsu massage, from Japan, in which the therapist applies pressure at various points of the body; Thai massage, which sometimes involves stretching; and Marma massage, from the Ayurvedic tradition of India, which involves a mixture of slow, gentle strokes and brisk, invigorating movements.

Exercise

Exercise can often play an important role in helping patients tolerate cancer treatment. For many patients, exercise provides a heightened sense of vitality that improves their energy level and overall quality of life. Even light exercise can provide real benefits, and just taking a short stroll in the park can build strength as well as offer a moment of spiritual renewal. Walking up a single flight of stairs can provide an enhanced sense of self-sufficiency for a patient who only recently could not even get out of bed.

Biochemically, exercise helps the physiology in much the same way that turning the soil benefits a garden. Both the earth and the healthy cells of the human body need oxygen, and even slightly elevated rates of breathing and heart rate during exercise can help fulfill this need.

One of the most immediate and universal benefits of even brief periods of exercise is relief of stress and tension. This can be extremely helpful for patients, even if their endurance is limited by the effects of their disease or treatment. Studies have documented improvement in anxiety, depression, physical performance, and quality of life in cancer patients who exercise. Use common sense when considering any exercise program, and discuss any questions with your physician.

Yoga

Yoga is an almost magical technique for both the mind and the body. Although in the past yoga has been associated with difficult or strenuous postures, it is actually a gentle approach to creating awareness and ultimately union between the physical, mental, emotional, and spiritual aspects of ourselves. In fact, the word *yoga* is Sanskrit for "union."

Yoga exercises can be done by anyone at almost any time, even while lying in bed, sitting in a chair, or riding in a car. Elementary exercises are designed not to strain the body, but to stretch and tone the muscles and joints, increase energy, quiet the mind and breath, and promote greater awareness and inner calm. Many patients feel deeply renewed and rejuvenated after a yoga session, and there is evidence that yoga can enhance many physiologic processes of the body, including immune function, digestion, circulation, and sleep.

Relaxation

Long periods of worry and harried activity, whether physical, mental, or emotional, are bound to impede the healing process. Few things can counteract this more effectively than deep relaxation. Thus, it is absolutely vital that time be set aside for this on the journey through cancer. The kind of relaxation I am referring to here does *not* include watching television, reading books or magazines, or talking with family or friends, because in all these activities your mind remains active. Deep relaxation is a process that involves consciously entering into a state in which the body, mind, and heart become quiet and tranquil, and are restored on a profound level.

Relaxation is one of the important components of healing that patients and family members tend to overlook. While overlooking it is certainly understandable in the context of cancer treatment and its many demands, I believe it is unfortunate. Healing on many levels is profoundly facilitated by deep relaxation. Aspects of healing are accessed in deep relaxation that are experienced nowhere else. It is one of the simplest yet most powerful, direct, and accessible things that a patient can do to consciously help themselves on their journey.

There are many ways to facilitate deep relaxation and to make it easier and more enjoyable, including guided relaxation tapes, inspirational pieces of music, yoga, or a variety of meditation techniques. The benefits from all these techniques are immediate, diverse, and long-lasting.

Journaling

At various times throughout history, keeping a journal was a widespread and important part of daily life. Instinctively, many people discovered that they felt better after writing about the events in their lives and their innermost thoughts, feelings, and impressions. This remains true today—and though there are a large number of journal writers at the present time, it is only recently that the health-related benefits of journaling have been scientifically documented.

Several studies in the medical literature have explored the measurable benefits of writing about events in one's life, including improved immune function and overall health. A 1999 article published in the *Journal of the American Medical Association* discussed an intriguing study in which asthma and rheumatoid arthritis patients were found to have significantly reduced symptoms after writing about stressful events in their lives for twenty minutes a day over a period of several days. These improvements were beyond those attributable to the standard medical care that all the participants received.

Although the medical issues of cancer are unique, and obviously different from those of asthma or arthritis, there is no doubt that putting your thoughts and feelings into writing can have significant emotional benefits on the journey through cancer. I encourage all of my patients—and their loved ones—to purchase a hard-bound journal and spend some time each day writing in it. Even five or ten minutes a day is helpful.

Journaling on a consistent basis provides an outlet for completely honest, unfiltered expression of yourself that is available to you at all times. It provides a record of your thoughts, questions, and experiences that may surprise and inspire you in the future. It also provides a reference to draw upon during difficult moments and a place to record important milestones. Finally, it gives you a precious opportunity to contact that part of yourself that is the silent witness of all the events in your life.

Visualization and Guided Imagery

Visualization and guided imagery are two related techniques that have gained great acceptance among cancer patients over the last twenty years. In both techniques, patients typically lie in a comfortable position with their eyes closed for a period of time. Patients are guided through the process by a facilitator, or they can do it on their own.

In visualization, patients intentionally create specific images in their mind's eye to facilitate healing. Examples include visualizing "Pac men" or "knights in shining armor" destroying cancer cells throughout the body, or visualizing cancer cells dissolving into nothingness. The biochemical helpfulness of this technique remains controversial, but there is no doubt that patients benefit when negative thoughts are replaced by images of strength and empowerment. I prefer patients to visualize their bodies filled with love, light, and healing energy, but if someone chooses to imagine an army destroying cancer cells, I support them in doing so.

Guided imagery is similar to visualization, but it often includes a script or narrative that is read by a facilitator or played on an audiotape. The narrative often involves guiding the patient's consciousness to scenes or places of serenity and peace, such as tranquil gardens, healing meadows, or a soft and gentle seashore. In these settings, the patient gains access to inner wisdom, guidance, intuition, and reserves of powerful healing energy within. A variety of outstanding guided imagery tapes are available that can help patients deal more effectively with specific concerns, such as fear, anxiety, depression, or even the side effects of chemotherapy. A list of some excellent guided imagery tapes is provided in Appendix 1.

Acupuncture

Acupuncture, an ancient healing technique that originated in China, has been increasingly accepted and utilized in the West over the last twenty years. In the practice of acupuncture, extremely thin, sterile needles are carefully placed by the acupuncturist at specific points on the patient's body to facilitate the natural flow of vital energy, called *chi*.

In China, acupuncture has been used for centuries as a successful treatment for a wide variety of ailments. In the West, it is becoming understood that acupuncture has many valuable applications for medicine in general, and for cancer patients in particular. Acupuncture can be helpful in relieving symptoms such as pain, fatigue, insomnia, and muscle and joint aches. In 1998, acupuncture was recognized by the National Institutes of Health as a proven, effective treatment for chemotherapy-related nausea and vomiting. Acupuncture is also an excellent way to mobilize subtle levels of energy throughout the entire body, promoting overall healing and wellness.

Chiropractic

In the United States, chiropractic is one of the most widely utilized forms of complementary medicine. It has proven value in treating back, neck, and shoulder pain, particularly when caused by misaligned vertebrae. By reestablishing proper alignment of the entire vertebral column, proper function of the vast network of nerves that extend from the spinal cord to all the organs of the body is facilitated. Chiropractic promotes not only pain relief but overall health and vitality.

For all its acknowledged benefits, chiropractic must be used with special care by cancer patients who may have bone metastases. As with other complementary modalities, it is important to discuss the use of chiropractic with your physician before proceeding.

Homeopathy

Homeopathy is a system of medicine that was founded in the eighteenth century by the German physician Samuel Hahnemann. It is widely accepted in Europe, and in recent years has been gaining recognition in the United States.

Homeopathy is based on the principle that illnesses are specific to individuals and that "like cures like." Homeopathic remedies are composed of minute amounts of substances that, in larger amounts, would cause the very same symptoms that a patient is currently experiencing. The theoretical basis of vaccines is similar. In homeopathy, however, the substances are sequentially diluted with pure water or alcohol, almost to the point of disappearance. This is based on another homeopathic principle: remedies *gain* potency the more they are diluted.

Remedies are prescribed by a homeopathic physician after an extensive interview process and are highly specific for the individual. Although the precise mechanism of action of homeopathic remedies is not scientifically understood, many patients report significant responses and benefits. Homeopathic remedies may be particularly useful for cancer patients in dealing with a variety of symptoms, including depression, anxiety, insomnia, loss of appetite, and treatment-related nausea and vomiting, among others.

Therapeutic Touch

Therapeutic Touch combines insights of ancient healing practices such as "laying on of hands" and contemporary theories of energy transfer drawn from physics and neurochemistry. The modern system of Therapeutic Touch was organized by Dolores Krieger, a professor of nursing at New York University. Therapy sessions include procedures to focus the therapist's attention on the patient, assessment of underlying energy imbalances in the patient's body, and finally rebalancing the patient's energy field. To accomplish this, the therapist passes his or her hands, held two to six inches over the patient's body, down the length of the body, past the toes, and out of the body. Sessions usually last twenty to thirty minutes, and conclude with the practitioner transferring energy to the patient to further promote healing at all levels.

Reiki Therapy

Reiki is an ancient healing technique brought to prominence in Japan during the nineteenth century. Reiki therapy uses touch to stimulate the body's inner healing energy, but it is not simply a physiological procedure. Rather, it is a spiritual modality whose effectiveness is based on love and inner wisdom rather than clinical diagnosis and treatment. Reiki practitioners are trained by masters to perform the technique and teach it to others over a short period of time. Although therapy sessions may last for an hour or more, Reiki is not a difficult or esoteric therapy. It can be easily learned and used by patients themselves, and this is part of its appeal.

ALTERNATIVE MEDICINE

The use of alternative forms of cancer treatment is a source of great concern and confusion for patients and oncologists alike. Many different forms of alternative cancer therapies exist, often with openly conflicting theoretical bases. None of them have undisputed, scientifically proven benefit. Almost all require significant out-of-pocket expenses. Many have hidden costs and potential risks. And yet their appeal remains broad and understandable, particularly in the face of a potentially life-threatening illness.

In his outstanding and highly informative 1994 book, *Choices in Healing,* Michael Lerner makes many valuable and important observations regarding so-called alternative or unproven cancer therapies. Among his observations are the following:

• Lerner states he saw "no decisive and scientifically documented cure for any type of cancer among the unconventional therapies."

• Lerner suggests that patients must distinguish between the "plausibility of the therapy itself, the credibility and character of the practitioner, and the quality of the service itself." Highly ethical and charismatic healers may sincerely believe in treatments that have no scientific basis. Often the treatments are available only in certain hard-to-reach locations, and these may be outside the United States. Patients may be eager to receive the treatments despite the difficulties involved, simply because of their own desperation or the convincing presentation of the provider. This can be a dangerous situation for patients who may already be weakened by cancer.

• Lerner describes a psychological phenomenon in which "an inverse relationship exists between the openness of the alternative pharmacological therapies and the level of public interest in the therapy." In other words, the more exotic and esoteric the treatment, the greater the mystique in the minds of some patients. The idea of a conspiracy on the part of the government or pharmaceutical companies to suppress cures for cancer has a long and colorful history. As with political conspiracy theories, this line of thinking appeals to people who feel their urgent needs are not being met by the establishment. But choosing treatments based on anger or frustration with mainstream medicine can be a perilous course.

These are important considerations, but I don't intend them to be a global, unqualified rejection of alternative therapies. High-dose vitamins, Essiac tea, Laetrile, and other treatments have been described by numerous patients as being beneficial. In the absence of proof to the contrary, it is reasonable to assume that, for some patients, this may indeed have been true. Some patients even believe they have been cured by alternative therapies. As implausible as this may seem from a conventional viewpoint, this too may have occurred on occasion. It is important to remember that our approach to cancer can change at any time with a new discovery or a completely unanticipated form of treatment. Such things have happened repeatedly in the history of medicine. At the present time, alternative therapies have *not* been proven effective in accordance with the definitions of scientific medicine. While some therapies may have value or benefit, the magnitude and reliability of that benefit is still unknown. Currently, it seems relatively small, at best, and some of the therapies may actually be harmful. All too often, their utilization can cause a patient to forgo a potentially life-saving proven treatment.

To illustrate some of the issues that arise with unproven cancer therapies, it is helpful to look at a well-known case in point: shark cartilage.

It is an interesting fact of the natural world that sharks rarely get cancer. Despite, or perhaps because they are one of the oldest surviving forms of animal life, something about shark biology seems to resist development of malignant tumors. What, then, are the implications of this anomaly for the treatment of human cancer? Or, are there *any* implications?

From the observation that sharks rarely get cancer, a multimillion-dollar industry of books, Web sites, and shark-based medicines has developed—despite the absence of any reliable, scientifically proven benefit to cancer patients. One of the claims for shark cartilage is that it works by inhibiting the growth of tumor-supporting blood vessels. In medical terminology, this is known as *anti-angiogenesis* (from the Greek *angio,* meaning blood vessel, and *genesis,* meaning to form). Anti-angiogenesis is an active area of mainstream cancer research. Laboratory tests have revealed that cartilage from sharks and other animals can inhibit the development of blood vessels under experimental conditions. However, positive results in laboratory tests, even assuming they can withstand the scrutiny of scientific review, by no means guarantee a viable anticancer treatment in humans.

The history of oncology is filled with stories of potential cancer cures that reportedly worked well in laboratory animals or petri dishes, but failed in human subjects. In the case of shark cartilage, there are many reasons why a similar scenario would occur.

For example, shark cartilage treatments are usually administered orally. As with food and other substances, ingesting shark cartilage powder should lead to the enzymatic breakdown of the very proteins that are purportedly the active ingredient of the treatment. Thus many scientists believe it is extremely unlikely that any anti-angiogenesis factors present in the cartilage would be absorbed into the bloodstream in amounts sufficient to effect any activity against tumors. A second claim regarding the activity of shark cartilage is that it functions as an "immune stimulant." However, no scientific evidence for this exists. Even if it were true, stimulation of the immune system by natural substances has rarely, if ever, been an effective means of cancer treatment.

Only limited clinical studies of shark cartilage have been performed, with mixed results. One study, performed under careful, scientific conditions and reported in the *Journal of Clinical Oncology* in November 1998, involved sixty patients with a variety of previously treated, advanced cancers who were given oral doses of shark cartilage as their only therapy. After twelve weeks of therapy, no patient achieved a complete or even partial remission. Ten patients showed no progression in their cancer over the duration of their treatment. To mainstream researchers, this observation was not significant, since many cancers do not progress consistently or rapidly. But to people predisposed to believe in shark cartilage, it was a highly significant development. Unwilling to accept the negative results of the study, shark cartilage advocates also criticized the types of patients selected for the study, the quality of the shark cartilage that was used, and the way it was administered.

Perhaps only repeated, overwhelming scientific evidence will dissuade fervent believers in alternative therapies. In the past, rigorous studies of many of these treatments have only reluctantly been undertaken by mainstream medicine or been allowed by the adherents of alternative therapies. Fortunately, this situation is now changing. In 1992, under mandate from the United States Congress, the National Institutes of Health established the Office of Alternative Medicine (OAM) as a resource for research on alternative forms of medicine. In 1998, the OAM was expanded into the National Center for Complementary and Alternative Medicine (NCCAM), in order to "facilitate the evaluation of alternative medical treatment modalities" and determine their effectiveness.

Scientific studies of different alternative forms of cancer therapy are now under way, with increasing frequency. Until the results of these and future studies are available, and clear guidelines for the safe and appropriate utilization of specific alternative therapies has been established, I recommend that patients use them with great caution, and only if no scientifically proven therapies are available to help them.

EASTERN HEALING TRADITIONS

Ayurveda

The traditional life science of India is one of the world's oldest and most comprehensive healing systems, and has been practiced for over three thousand years. Ayurveda, which means the "science of life" in Sanskrit, perceives the universe as a whole—and human beings in particular—as a dynamic interplay of three principles that pervade all levels of creation. These principles, called *doshas,* exist in all living things, and are called *vata, pitta,* and *kapha.* They correspond to specific metabolic functions in the body, as well as to more fundamental forces of nature.

Good health depends upon maintaining a balance of the doshas that is appropriate for each individual. Ayurveda understands disease as a deviation from this natural state of balance and provides an interesting alternative to the Western mechanical model of illness. When a patient is sick, the Ayurvedic physician seeks to identify the underlying cause and nature of the dosha imbalance, and offers a variety of natural therapies that are specifically tailored for the individual. These therapies are intended not only to relieve symptoms but, more important, to restore the doshas to their natural state of balance, thus restoring health.

As an eminently practical and inclusive approach to sickness and health, Ayurveda makes use of herbal supplements, yoga and meditation, and cleansing techniques designed to clear toxins from the body as well as eliminate destructive impulses from the mind and spirit. One of the most profound aspects of Ayurveda is its understanding that physical health is not an end in itself. According to legend, the ancient physicians who formulated Ayurveda did so with the understanding that the pain and suffering of disease could impede life's deeper purpose, which is spiritual realization. Once the physical body is healed, we can begin to achieve our full spiritual potential.

Traditional Chinese Medicine

Traditional Chinese Medicine dates back nearly three thousand years and is still used by one-fifth of the world's population. While the Western idea of longevity refers fundamentally to length of life, in the Chinese medical tradition longevity includes what the West calls "quality of life," so merely living for many years is meaningless without health, vitality, and joy.

It is a principle of Chinese Medicine that illness arises from disruptions in the flow of *chi*, or life energy, within the body. Under conditions of good health, chi flows naturally through an extensive network of invisible channels, or *meridians*, that flow through the body and connect all of the internal organs and glands. Disruptions of the flow of chi can occur from blockages in the meridians caused by a variety of mechanical or physiological processes in the body. Chi can also flow in amounts that are excessive or deficient, thus contributing to illness.

Traditional Chinese Medicine recognizes two complementary but opposing qualities of the universe, *yin* and *yang*. These principles correspond to polarities observable throughout nature, including male and female, hot and cold, and day and night.

Yin and yang are central to both diagnosis and treatment in Chinese medicine. Certain illnesses are associated with yin, while others are considered yang disorders. The five elements (fire, earth, metal, water, and wood) also play an important role in health and disease. Imbalances in yin, and yang, as well as in the five elements, cause disruptions to the flow of chi, and disease results.

To restore proper balance in the body, Chinese Medicine uses herbal preparations, massage, *moxibustion* (the burning of special herbs over particular points of the body), cupping, energy exercises *(qigong),* meditation, and acupuncture. Like Ayurveda, Traditional Chinese Medicine is a highly evolved and coherent approach that emphasizes treating the whole person rather than focusing on the particular illness. This is true for the Chinese medicine approach to cancer, as well as other diseases. A large body of research exists on the use of Chinese herbs in cancer, either as primary therapy or in combination with more conventional treatments. Most of this research has been performed in China, and it is now attracting increasing attention in the West.

Tibetan Medicine

The origins of the 1,300-year-old science of Tibetan Medicine are rooted in the teachings of the Buddha, which emphasize the intimate relationship between body and mind. In the central text of Tibetan Medicine, called the *rGyud bzi,* or the *Four Tantras,* physical disease is understood to originate, ultimately, from one primary cause: ignorance of our true nature. From this fundamental ignorance arises what are called the "three poisons" of desire, hatred, and confusion. Over time, these three poisons cause disturbances in three fundamental energy systems of the body, called *lung, tripa,* and *badken* (the three *nyepa*). These disturbances ultimately manifest as physical illness.

As in Ayurveda and Traditional Chinese Medicine, Tibetan doctors endeavor to understand the cause and nature of the imbalances that are causing the patient's problems, and then to restore them to proper balance. Tibetan diagnosis relies upon extensive questioning of the patient, physical examination, examination of the tongue, urinalysis, and an extremely elaborate method of analyzing the pulse. In combination, these yield exquisitely detailed information about the underlying physiologic as well as mental and emotional conditions of the patient. The physician then prescribes a variety of natural remedies intended to restore harmony and balance to the three *nyepa*.

Tibetan medicines are largely based on combinations of herbs but can also contain animal products or even precious gems or metals. Dietary changes, physical exercises, moxibustion, cleansing practices, and a Tibetan form of acupuncture may also be prescribed. Finally, a variety of spiritual practices are recommended if appropriate to facilitate even deeper levels of healing. By combining sharply focused clinical knowledge with profound spiritual understanding and intention, Tibetan Medicine provides an extraordinary model for individual health care as well as for Western medicine as a whole.

Some Practical Suggestions

There are so many things you can do to nurture the garden of your body. The suggestions below are just a preliminary list, and you can surely come up with more. A useful guiding principle is to think of your body as a garden that needs sunlight, water, oxygen, nourishment, and loving care and attention. Once you've embraced this idea, exercise is no longer just a matter of physical exertion, it is an opportunity for bringing oxygen to the deep soil of your being. Similarly, eating nutritious, healthful food is no longer done simply to prevent or eliminate cancer; it is a way to fertilize and nourish the garden of the self. In all your activities, try to remain aware of this powerful and profound metaphor. When you keep the idea of your body as a garden in the forefront of your consciousness, you will naturally begin to live in ways that ensure your garden's continuing healthy growth.

- Look at your diet. Are you eating healthy foods every day? Refer to the nutrition guidelines listed on page 99.
- Eat foods that you enjoy. Try to become aware of the difference between satisfying a momentary craving for a particular food and eating something that is genuinely nourishing and satisfying to you—and your body.
- Consider giving yourself the gift of a massage at least once a week, more if you are able.

- Begin an exercise program, but use common sense. If you are tired, consider a simple walk for a few minutes each day, or for a longer time if comfortable.
- Join a yoga class. Experience the joys of gentle stretching and deep relaxation.
- Drink 6–8 glasses of spring water a day. Remember, it is important to water the garden of your being daily if you want it to be healthy.
- Make sure that your bowels are moving regularly. Eliminating toxins from your body is very important. If you are having any difficulties in this area, discuss it immediately with your physician.
- Breathe deeply for ten breaths, at least three times a day. Inhale for a count of two, hold for a count of eight, and exhale for a count of four. On the exhalation, push all of the air out of your lungs. This will deeply oxygenate your blood, improve the flow of lymph throughout the body, and help you to relax, think more clearly, and become more focused.
- Consider seeing an acupuncturist for a general evaluation.
- Explore the benefits of Therapeutic Touch, Reiki therapy, or other forms of energy healing.
- Remember that the garden of your being needs sunshine! Spend some time each day in nature. Even if you live in a city, take at least a few minutes a day to appreciate the sun, the sky, and whatever trees and plants are around you.
- Get a hard-bound journal, and spend at least five to ten minutes a day writing down your thoughts, feelings, and impressions. Keep a record of important events, questions, ideas, or inspirations that come to you as well.
- Take time every day to rest and relax. Explore the benefits of deep relaxation on a consistent basis.
- Try some guided imagery tapes and discover new resources of healing, creativity, intuition, and inner wisdom.

7

LEVEL FOUR:
EMOTIONAL HEALING

WE SHALL NOT CEASE FROM EXPLORATION. AND
THE END OF ALL OUR EXPLORING WILL BE TO
ARRIVE WHERE WE STARTED, AND KNOW THE
PLACE FOR THE FIRST TIME.

                                        —T.S. ELIOT

An important transition takes place between Levels Three and Four of this program. So far our principal focus has been on the biological and clinical issues of the journey through cancer. We've explored the major issues involved in understanding cancer types, staging, and treatment, as well as the importance of having trust in your doctor—including his or her personal and spiritual qualities as well as technical expertise. We've looked at our common, human instinct and need for connection with others, and the important benefits that can be derived from a variety of psychosocial support programs. And we've considered an entirely new way of perceiving our body—*as a garden, rather than a machine*—and begun to explore the vast array of alternative and complementary therapies that can help facilitate nurturing and healing.

Now the healing intention turns inward. Many patients never make this shift in focus. When that happens, I believe that they have missed an important opportunity.

Any challenge in life—and especially a great challenge like cancer—can ignite the mind and heart to search for deeper understanding. Once you have made the decision to put your medical care in the hands of a trusted physician, you are then free to devote attention to any underlying human issues that may be unresolved but that will certainly affect your healing process. Now the journey through cancer becomes less about cells, chemicals, and diets, and more about thoughts and feelings.

Remarkably, an interesting paradox now appears. By turning some of your attention away from the clinical issues of care, you may actually increase the effectiveness of your treatment.

When cancer has been detected in the lung, breast, colon, or any other vital organ, medicine often fails to recognize that the heart is always involved as well. Here I am referring not to the physical pump located in the middle of the chest, but rather to the emotional and spiritual center of every human being. This metaphorical heart is invariably affected and often transformed by a cancer diagnosis. If that transformation is a positive one, true healing can take place at every level of being.

Robots or machines do not get cancer. Living and breathing human beings develop malignant cells in their bodies and respond to the disease with thoughts and feelings that are a mix of chemistry, psychology, genetics, and the mysterious nature of consciousness itself. The interplay of all these factors in the journey through cancer is an authentic expression of the human condition: at times painful and frustrating, at other times heroic and inspirational, but always a mystery to behold. One thing, though, is absolutely certain. All cancer patients, as well as everyone close to them, will be exposed to a seemingly infinite variety of emotions along the way.

Trying to ignore or deny those feelings is fundamentally self-destructive. It only strengthens the repressed emotions and makes it more likely that they will eventually break through with doubled force. Make no mistake: cancer is an emotional roller-coaster ride. There are times when you'll want to scream, and there are times when you'll want to cry. Incredible as it may seem, there are even times when you'll want to laugh.

After serving as physician, friend, coach, mentor, and guide for thousands of patients and their family members over many years, I can say that *not one single person* has ever truly healed from cancer without undergoing a transformation and healing of their emotional self. This is a key point, and I want to make it clearly. The challenges encountered in the diagnosis and treatment of cancer are often intense and profound. The rigors of the journey are such that inner vulnerabilities can be laid bare and even exacerbated. Addressing these very real, understandable, and human vulnerabilities—and everything that often accompanies them—is therefore of vital importance.

THE EMOTIONAL PARADIGM

For most people, the flood of practical questions encountered during the initial phase of cancer treatment does eventually subside. When that happens, complex and often uncomfortable feelings can begin to assert themselves, and decisions have to be made about how to deal with them. Sometimes the feelings are completely ignored, sometimes they're completely indulged, but they are almost always misunderstood unless they're given conscious attention. The roller coaster of feelings can have some steep ups and downs, for which few people are prepared. Fear is only the most obvious and accessible emotion associated with cancer. I've seen a full spectrum of rage, resentment, frustration, sadness, guilt, remorse, doubt, and discouragement in virtually everyone who has tried to deal with cancer, including myself, during my father's illness. At the very least, these emotions deserve to be acknowledged. The real challenge, however, is working through them, and finding release and freedom from them in a safe and positive way.

Many patients actively bottle up their emotional responses to their illness. So often I've walked into exam rooms and found cancer patients trying with all their might to present themselves as cool, calm, and collected. Unresolved emotions are often expressed as irritation, impatience, and annoyance at even being in the presence of the doctor. All sorts of silent messages are beamed my way:

> *This shouldn't be happening. I resent it. I won't stand for it. I'm a CEO, and I'm used to being in charge.*

> *I'm not going to let anyone see I'm upset by this. Not you, and especially not my husband.*

> *Money is no object to me. I've always been able to buy my way out of anything, and I'll buy my way out of this, too.*

But perhaps the most common message comes from the vast majority of patients who must deal with the significant logistical challenges of cancer, including day care for children, time off from work, and financial pressures. For these people, the impulse to suppress their emotions has a different rationale:

I just don't have time for this. I've got more important things to do.

I don't have time to worry about my feelings.

As we begin the consultation, conversations with patients who are responding in this way are often stiff and abrupt. The focus is on getting rid of the problem and attending to other business. However, after completing the history and physical examination, I make a point of gently asking, "How are you feeling in all this, Mr. Jones? What's this really been like for you, Mrs. Smith?" Again and again, these simple questions trigger dramatic outpourings of emotion. In a heartbeat, Mr. Jones and Mrs. Smith become lost and lonely children, weeping uncontrollably. Deep pain and frustration, often suppressed for years, instantly rises to the surface.

For me, the saddest thing is how quickly patients who respond like this seek to reestablish the internal status quo. Men straighten their ties, women redo their lipstick and makeup—and they depart *as if nothing had happened!* The feelings are so troubling that they must never be shown to the world—or even acknowledged. Yet, by denying their emotions, patients often deprive themselves of the very experience of healing that they are really seeking when they come to me for help.

It is also unfortunate that mainstream medicine minimizes the importance of emotional work in the healing process. A major reason for this is that, with the exception of psychiatrists, doctors are not trained, honored, or paid to adequately address the emotional concerns of cancer patients and family members. Furthermore, distinguishing emotional factors that are functional and situational from those that are derived from an underlying neurochemical imbalance can be a subtle, complex, and time-consuming process. Depression—which occurs in *up to 50 percent of cancer patients*—may be mistaken for anxiety, or vice versa. Genuine and appropriate grieving is often tagged as depression and is frequently overmedicated or undermedicated. A number of factors contribute to this, including the training, experience, and practice habits of the physician, as well as the patient's wishes and willingness to explore and disclose their true feelings.

THE ELEPHANT IN THE ROOM

In some respects, cancer is like an elephant that suddenly appears in your living room. Certainly the first order of business is to get the elephant out, but that may take some time. Meanwhile, what should you do? Some people block everything out of their lives except the elephant. They don't think or talk about anything else. Other people try to pretend the elephant isn't there: "Elephant? What elephant?"

The best answer to such an urgent but unwieldy problem lies somewhere between the two extremes. Once you give yourself permission to deal appropriately with the emotional issues associated with your illness, you can become freed from the burdens that accompany both denial and preoccupation.

In helping people make the journey through cancer, one of my greatest priorities is to skillfully and gently help patients address and resolve the feelings that must be dealt with. If this doesn't happen, whether their tumor shrinks or even goes into complete remission, genuine healing will not have occurred. In an important way, the damage done by cancer will still be present. In fact, it will always be present until hidden emotional pain is brought out in the light of awareness and healed in the light of love.

When I first met Laura Hill and her husband, Steve, they had been dealing with Laura's metastatic breast cancer for four years. Laura was a bright, fifty-one-year-old woman who originally presented with Stage II disease and had undergone a modified radical mastectomy and axillary lymph node dissection, followed by adjuvant chemotherapy and tamoxifen. A year later, however, her cancer returned, and was found in her lungs, liver, and on her chest wall. She went through high-dose chemotherapy with stem cell support at a major cancer center, with excellent results. Soon thereafter, however, her cancer once again came back. There followed several rounds of "salvage chemotherapy," repeated radiation therapy treatments to her chest wall, and a variety of hormonal therapies for breast cancer. The disease always reappeared.

Laura and Steve started to lose faith in mainstream approaches. They began to spend their life savings traveling to treatment centers and holistic healing facilities in America, Mexico, and the Bahamas, searching desperately for a cure. Laura underwent diet therapies, cleansing programs, coffee enemas, high-dose intravenous vitamin infusions, shark cartilage, Essiac tea, and mistletoe extract. Nothing worked, although one practitioner after another promised relief from the assault of her cancer. Whenever it became clear that a new therapy was not working, Laura and Steve would be off to the next healing center, shaman, sweat lodge, herbalist, homeopath, chiropractor, naturopath, or acupuncturist. Laura was rolfed, rebirthed, and energy balanced, and her chakras were repeatedly aligned. Exotic crystals were placed on every part of her body, and she visualized her cancer cells being eaten by white knights in shining armor a million times. Nothing worked.

Laura and Steve came to see me through a friend's recommendation. I was described as a board-certified oncologist who also understood and appreciated the value of other healing methods and traditions, someone who would give Laura chemotherapy if I believed it could help her, and who would honor and support her desire to do everything possible to help herself live.

After their long, lonely ordeal, Steve and Laura were deeply discouraged but not yet ready to give up hope. They loved each other. They loved their two kids. They loved life and they wanted more time together. They weren't ready for her to die.

But they were frustrated, and they were angry at so many things— especially at the cancer that had destroyed the life they had known together. They were also angry about how they'd been treated at conventional cancer centers, and how they'd been ridiculed for wanting to explore other options. Yet they also felt they'd been misled at alternative healing centers, even if by sincere and well-intentioned people.

Laura and Steve came to my office with a box of medical records, the sad chronicle of two people fighting against a formidable challenge. As I sifted through the records, I admired their courage and determination. Even in coming to see me, they were willing to risk yet more disappointment because of their desire for Laura to live.

We began to talk, and I asked to hear their story in their own words. Laura spoke first, then Steve took over. They had reiterated the story many times and had become a well-synchronized team in narrating their experiences. I had the feeling that Laura was growing tired of talking about it. Steve, on the other hand, was intent on recounting every incident, every disappointment. In retelling the story, he became animated, angry, and even sarcastic and contemptuous about the people they had met. Before long he even became hostile to me, someone he had never met before, a doctor to whom he had brought his wife for help.

Soon Steve was almost yelling. "They told her this, and they told her that, and nothing worked! It's all bullshit! They tell her to take this chemo, or drink this tea, or do these enemas, or swallow these vitamins and minerals, and her cancer will go away! But it's lies! It's all lies! Nothing has worked!"

This was a man who had exhausted himself trying to save his wife's life. His love and devotion were so clear, but his frustration and despair was beginning to consume him.

Finally, silence. I asked Laura if I could examine her. As she removed her shirt, I saw lengths of gauze wound around her chest that were stained with blood, pus, and serum. Slowly, carefully, we began unwrapping the gauze together, revealing the disfigured body of a woman who had endured a truly heroic ordeal. Laura's right breast was gone, replaced by scar tissue. The underlying skin was thickened and discolored from the effects of radiation. Her right arm was puffed and swollen with lymphedema, and it was difficult for her to open and close her fist. Her left breast was also thickened, red, and swollen. Examining it more closely, I saw it was full of cancer. A small amount of blood was oozing from the nipple, and a mass of thick, red, nodular lesions—a number of which were also oozing blood and pus—covered her entire chest and extended around to the right side of her back.

Twice each day, Steve cleaned the wounds on Laura's chest, gave her antibiotics, and wrapped her with gauze. This had been going on for many months.

As I examined Laura, I recognized this as one of the most difficult cancer scenarios: the disease keeps reappearing, and nothing seems capable of making it "go away." Still, patients and their loved ones hunger for life.

Fortunately, several new chemotherapy drugs were now available that had a real chance of helping Laura on the clinical level—not to cure, but definitely to provide some relief from what her body was going through. However, there were many issues here beyond Laura's physical condition. It seemed to me that simply opening a discussion about more chemotherapy would have completely missed the point. The elephant seemed to be consuming all the air in the room. It would serve no one's interests to deny that fact by focusing only on her medical treatment or the purely clinical concerns.

After I finished examining Laura, she got dressed. I then turned to Steve and said, "May I ask you a question?"

"Sure," he replied.

"Have you and Laura talked very much about how you're feeling in all this?"

"What do you mean?"

"Well, I can see that both of you have become very knowledgeable about the relative strengths and weaknesses of various treatment options for breast cancer. I'm also deeply impressed by your courage and determination to keep fighting this disease. But along the way, have you and Laura taken the time to really talk in depth about what you're experiencing in this process? Have you communicated about what it's really like—with your doctors, or with yourselves?"

"No," Steve said, after a long silence. "Not really."

"Why not?"

Another long silence. Then: "There never seems to be time. There's always so much to do. And no one has ever asked us about those kinds of things. All they've ever talked about was what her next therapy should be."

I turned to his wife. "Laura, is that your experience too?"

Another long, sad silence. When Laura spoke at last, she expressed an almost universal perception among cancer patients: no one had ever really asked them how they *felt*, because the focus was always on *what they ought to do*. Consequently, they had devalued and lost touch with their feelings. This was clearly an issue that needed to be addressed as soon as possible. Any further discussion about "what they ought to do" clinically would be misdirected until we addressed the turbulent, underlying emotions that had been ignored for too long.

"Laura and Steve," I said, "I recognize that Laura's body most definitely needs love and attention and medical care right now, in a very serious way. And we can do a lot to help in this regard. But both of you also have minds and hearts and spirits, and these also need love and attention and care. If we focus only on the cancer, or on what new chemotherapy regimen to follow, or what herbs, vitamins, minerals, and supplements to take, we'll be bypassing really vast and important areas of the process, and I don't want to do it."

This shocked them a little bit. "What do you mean, 'I don't want to do it'?"

"Well, I'm not here simply to treat cancer, which is a very mechanical process. We can and will do an absolutely first-class, impeccable job with that—but it is *only one aspect of what needs to happen.* I'm also interested in seeing how I can help you both as human beings. But I can only do so much. You've got to get involved. You've got to participate, perhaps in a way you never have before. Are you willing to do that? Are you willing to start looking at the other dimensions of what is going on here as well? It may not be easy. Do you really want to do it?"

They were quiet for a while, and looked at each other silently. Then Laura asked, "Well, what's really involved?"

"A lot is involved, but we'll go slowly. We'll talk about everything, including what to do for your cancer. But we'll also talk about how you're really feeling deep in your hearts, and about what is really most important to you in life—what you really want to live for."

As I spoke these words, both Laura and Steve started to cry. I had seen this response in so many patients and family members when the door to hidden feelings began to open. After some time had passed I gently asked, "Why were you crying? Will you tell me?"

They answered almost in unison. The same answer I've heard over and over again: *"Because no one ever asked us how we're feeling."*

This was the beginning of a long and magical part of Laura and Steve's journey. In our talks over the coming days and weeks, by writing in their journals, and by participating in our support groups, much was discovered and much was healed. Steve had a chance to recognize and express his own anger and frustration at having his life, as well as Laura's, utterly consumed by her disease. "For four years," he cried, "I have focused completely on Laura and her needs. I have always had to put my own needs aside. Everyone in the family, all the doctors, all the healers— *everyone*—only focuses on Laura. For four years, it has always been 'What does Laura need today? What does Laura want today?' I love her so much, but I can't stand it anymore. What about me? Nobody says, 'Steve, what do *you* need today?' We haven't made love for over four years, and I miss it. I feel frustrated and angry. I also feel lonely, and so sad. And then, when I hear myself say things like this, I feel so guilty. How can I feel pity for myself? Look at what she has had to go through. I should be ashamed of myself to complain. I am ashamed of my selfishness, and ashamed that I haven't been able to save her. Isn't that what a husband is supposed to do? I've tried everything I can, but it is never good enough. Despite everything I've tried to do, her cancer keeps coming back, and I can't save her. I feel like a failure. I've given everything I have, but in the end I couldn't save my beloved wife and friend."

Slowly, Laura also began to reveal her deepest emotions, which were just as powerful.

"I feel so tired, and so afraid. I'm not sure I can keep on going like this anymore, but I'm petrified to admit it. I'm afraid Steve will hate me if I say a part of me wants to give up. Look at all he's done for me. How can I abandon him? I would feel so guilty. In fact, I *already* feel guilty. This cancer has disrupted everything in our lives. Steve has had to give up so much to keep me going. It has nearly wiped us out financially. If I die, what will Steve have left? What will be left to give to our kids? I'm also mad, *really mad*, because this cancer has robbed me of so much, too. We worked so hard to have a life together, to raise our kids and then have fun, and it has all been lost. There were so many things I wanted to do and experience. Look at me, I'm not a woman any longer. I'm not even sure I'm a person any longer. I used to look great. I had great breasts, and a great body. Men were always attracted to me. Now, no one would ever think of coming near me. Even Steve won't come near me anymore— except to change my bandages. Who can call this living? I'm also mad at Steve because he won't ever leave me alone. All day long he is asking me, what do I want, what can he get me, what can he do for me. I just want him to stop sometimes, and leave me alone. Sometimes I just want to be left alone and cry. But I can't say it because he will feel hurt and abandoned, and I don't want to hurt him. I love him so much. I'm so lucky to have him, but I'm also so mad at him. He mopes and feels sorry for himself, and he thinks I don't know. How dare he feel sorry for himself? I'm the one with cancer, not him. At times I am so furious at him for this, and then I feel guilty again. Oh God, I don't know how I can handle it all!"

As I watched Laura and Steve acknowledge and explore these feelings, my admiration for them, and my love for them, deepened even more. As they gave themselves permission to experience their feelings without judgment, and as they learned ways of expressing their feelings without attacking or blaming each other, their relationship began to blossom and expand as never before. They realized that they were human, and that all their feelings and emotions were understandable, and so deeply human. They also began to realize that even though they had these feelings, the feelings were *not who they really are*. Even though the emotional waves could at times rage fiercely, there was a deeper part of themselves, and their love for each other, that was safe, protected, and untouched by it all. As they continued on this process of self-discovery and self-disclosure, they moved deeper and deeper into one of the most profound experiences of love and forgiveness that a human can have. They learned to *completely forgive themselves,* and *accept and embrace themselves for who they are.* And then they slowly began to *forgive each other,* and *forgive everyone they felt had ever "wronged" them in their lives.* Slowly, one by one, the overwhelming burdens of guilt, shame, anger, rage, and resentment began to lift, and they could focus on the gifts they still had for each other and the love they still had to share.

Laura and Steve shared another nine months together, and then she died. Those months were not always easy, but they were rich and precious, and filled with great discoveries, growth, healing, and love.

It is time for medicine to pay attention to the elephants in the room that are so often completely ignored in the urgent drama of clinical cancer care. Helping patients and families face the emotional issues of cancer—

whatever they are, whatever form they may take, and wherever they may lead—must be one of our highest priorities as caregivers. In the life-or-death context of cancer treatment, doctors, patients, and deeply concerned family members may have difficulty with my emphasis on addressing emotional issues. But seeing cancer only in terms of biochemistry and physiology is a gross oversimplification and a disservice to everyone. When I urge patients to direct their focus away from the specific details of their diagnosis and their treatment modalities, I'm not asking them to avoid or deny the serious issues of the cancer experience. Rather, I'm suggesting that the *really* serious issues encompass a much wider universe than they may have realized—and that *all* those issues must be carefully and fully addressed in order for healing to take place at the deepest levels.

Because these emotions can be so intense, and because they're often difficult to separate from the physical dimensions of the illness, emotional healing requires insight, tact, and great sensitivity from all involved. The process is often easier to recognize than it is to define. There is also no "magic formula" for putting it into practice. But here is a true story that shows how it works.

One Saturday I went to see David Buchanan on my usual morning hospital rounds. He was a kind, courageous, forty-two-year-old man with AIDS who had spent the better part of the previous nine months battling Kaposi's sarcoma (KS). In the first decade of the AIDS epidemic KS was quite common, and David had a particularly severe case. He had a number of KS lesions scattered around his body, but his legs in particular had become so extensively involved that they looked like two wet, swollen logs that had been burned and scorched in a fire with the bark left on. The skin from the tips of his toes to below both knees was blackened and purple, punctuated only by a number of pink open sores. He was in a lot of pain. *A lot* of pain. High doses of long-acting morphine given every eight hours barely kept him comfortable enough to lie still, and he couldn't even think about being able to stand or walk around. Although he hated to use a bedpan, day after day the bedside commode went untouched, barely two feet from his bed. Just two feet away, but it might as well have been on another planet.

His predicament that day was particularly discouraging because of all he had been through over the previous nine months. Remarkably, when I had first met him nine months earlier his legs had also looked like this. I'll never forget the day his partner wheeled him into my office for the first time with his legs propped up in a wheelchair. My heart sank as the bandages were cut away and I saw what they had been hiding. Extensive dermal-lymphatic invasion of KS was, at that time, one of the nastiest, most unyielding manifestations of AIDS. Unfortunately, I had seen it all too often, but David's legs were among the worst.

Over the next five months I saw David almost every week as we battled the KS in his legs. Quietly, fiercely, and without ever once complaining, he went through weeks of chemotherapy, radiation, and whirlpool treatments, followed by more chemotherapy. Little by little his legs got better, and then one day he shocked us all by walking proudly into the office on his own, announcing that he was here for his next treatment. He was limping badly and leaning on a cane, but for the first time in months he was walking on his own. Yippee! The whole office staff cheered, and many of us cried. We were so proud of him and so happy to see him walk again. It felt as though a miracle had happened in front of our eyes. We were even more surprised when he continued on with treatment and got even better. Eventually the skin on his legs started turning pink again and finally began to look like normal human legs.

Two months later he started having serious problems. Ten days after his last chemotherapy treatment his white blood cell counts plummeted. This had happened before, but they had always come right back up with Neupogen shots. This time he wasn't responding to Neupogen. Each day I held my breath as his counts remained low, and I prayed that the antibiotics he was taking would hold him over until his bone marrow recovered again. Late one afternoon, David called and told me that his temperature had suddenly spiked to 104 degrees, and he was feeling very sick. As I made arrangements for him to be admitted to the hospital, I knew he might be in for some real trouble. When he arrived at the hospital he couldn't breathe, and less than three hours later my worst fears were realized. He was in the ICU with bilateral pneumonia, respiratory failure, renal insufficiency, and profound sepsis. This was awful. Yesterday he had felt fine, but today he was in very real danger of dying. I was heartbroken. He had fought so hard and come so far.

Over the next few weeks he amazed us all once again. He fought back, little by little, "inch-by-inch, row-by-row," as the song goes. No matter what, he just wouldn't give up. Slowly, gradually, he continued to improve, and when he left the hospital more than six weeks later it felt as if we had witnessed another miracle.

The unfortunate thing was that during his time in the hospital we had not been able to give him any more treatment for his KS, and as a result his lesions had taken off again with a vengeance—like a bat out of hell, actually. His legs had once again become swollen and covered with the same, sickening darkness he had started out with nine months earlier. After all that work he was back to square one all over again. Just a few days after going home from the hospital, the pain in his legs became so unbearable that he had to be readmitted once again to get his pain under control and think about starting more treatment. He was also very sad, because in the midst of everything else his mother had died just the week before.

That is what was going on when I went into his room that Saturday morning to see him and try to cheer him up. The situation was complicated still further by the fact that I was not going to be able to give him great news about more treatment for his KS. I had spent a lot of time in the previous days trying to think of another chemotherapy regimen that we could use. His KS had already been treated with virtually every known active, available drug, and he had already received all the radiation his legs could tolerate. To top that off, he had nearly died from bone marrow failure and sepsis after his last cycle of chemotherapy.

"Good morning, David," I said quietly as I entered his room.

"Oh hi, Dr. Geffen," he replied. "Thank you for coming."

"How are you feeling today?" I asked.

"Well, okay, I guess. But my legs still hurt a lot. The morphine doesn't seem to do the trick like it used to."

I could see a great sadness and longing for rest in his big dark brown, battle-weary eyes. They seemed to stick out from his thin, bald head, his face now drawn and fatigued from chronic illness and pale from anemia and lack of sun.

In the nine months since we had met, it felt as if we had walked a million miles together. At each visit we always paused for just a second to silently acknowledge each other. It was always a precious moment, since neither of us knew how many more miles we had left to go.

"You know, Dr. Geffen," David said, "I'm a Christian, and I love Jesus very much. We've talked about this before. But lately I've been feeling that I must have failed in some way. That inside I must be impure."

"What do you mean, David?" I asked.

"Well," he said quietly, almost whispering, "look at what is happening to me. I've tried so hard to make up for my past, but it's not working. I think that Jesus must not have forgiven me for my sins."

His words stung my heart. David was one of the most beautiful, gentle, caring souls I had ever met, yet he felt that he had failed—not just with other people, but even with his savior. In my life I have come to understand and see again and again how, like nothing else, shame and self-hatred can destroy the human spirit and shatter dreams and lives. If ever there was a poison that could kill people more certainly than any cancer, or any sword, it was this. David's words carried the unmistakable tone of these most lethal destructive emotions. I felt sad and angry because I could see so clearly once again how shame and self-recrimination were helping to kill someone I cared for very much. Someone who was as gentle and loving as a soft breeze.

We talked about his feelings for a while. He had never opened up so deeply before or shared something this difficult. I was moved by his honesty, his vulnerability, and by his unspoken plea for help. I knew that we had to work on this or his healing would never be complete, regardless of what eventually happened to him. I asked him if he wanted to explore these feelings more deeply. I was relieved when he said, "Yes."

This was one of those moments that are both the true test and the true reward of an oncologist's life. At times like these, I feel humbled and privileged to enter into another person's reality. I am invited into that reality by their deep need and drawn toward it by my own wish to love and heal. It is not just a matter of guiding the patient, and certainly not of manipulating him or her in any way. Serving another human being—especially one with a fatal disease—involves allowing the false boundaries of ego, identity, and separation to melt and fall away. It involves giving the precious gift of your complete attention and focus, and merging so deeply in the heart that you become one. So much of modern medicine is a matter of turning dials, prescribing drugs, and reading charts and X rays. Moments like these, however, are also part of modern medicine—or at least they should be. They are what healers have experienced for thousands of years all over the world. This is where the scientific and the sacred meet, and where the apparent contradiction between them is revealed to be an illusion.

"David," I continued, "we've talked about your love of Jesus before, and your experience of Him. Do you really believe that He has not forgiven you for the things you feel you have done wrong in your life?"

David was silent for a long time. Finally, he replied.

"Actually, I *know* that He has forgiven me. But I don't *feel* it. I've never been able to feel it."

"Would you be willing to feel it right now?" I asked.

Again a pause, then, "Yes."

"Okay," I said, "close your eyes. I think we may be able to get this settled right here and now."

Still holding David's hand, I asked him to keep his eyes closed and see if he could picture Jesus standing in front of him.

He finally replied, "Yes."

"Okay, can you now feel Him in front of you as well?"

Again a long silence. Then, softly, "Yes."

"Good. Now, can you feel Him looking at you and can you feel His love for you?"

"Yes."

"Great. Now, David, I'd like you to look directly at Jesus and ask Him if He forgives you for everything you have ever done in your life that you feel was wrong. Okay? Are you able to do that right now?"

"No," he said. "I'm too scared."

"Okay," I replied, "it's okay. Just go slowly, and take your time. When you feel ready, go ahead and ask him if He forgives you. Do you think you might be able to do this now?"

"Yes," he whispered.

"Good. Now silently ask Him, and watch him closely."

I paused to allow this process to happen at its own pace. I wanted him to have a lot of time to have his own experience, without feeling rushed in any way. Eventually, though, I could tell David was having a hard time, so I asked, "Can you hear His reply?"

"No," David said, "I can't hear Him. I'm trying, but I can't hear Him. I want to, but I can't."

"Okay. Don't worry, just ask Him again silently, and listen with your heart. Just relax, and let Him speak to you in your heart."

This time David grew very quiet, and I could tell he was really asking now and really listening. I closed my eyes again and went deep into my own heart. I felt the presence of Jesus, Buddha, my own spiritual teachers, and all those beings throughout history who have given their lives to help relieve the suffering of humanity. I felt the presence of timeless awareness, and felt myself floating in and merged with the vast ocean of infinite love that is the essence of our true nature as humans. That which transcends and gives rise not only to the mind and the body but to all form, all creation, all phenomena. The bliss of this silence went on and on, until sometime later I finally heard David breathing more deeply than before. I opened my eyes and saw him begin to smile. He looked at me, and his big brown eyes were filled with big wet tears that rolled softly down his face.

My eyes instantly filled with tears, too. I hadn't seen him smile like this for so many weeks, and now he was actually glowing from within. His eyes sparkled with beams of light that filled the vast, timeless, silent space that surrounded and embraced us both.

As we looked at each other, blinking through our tears so we could keep seeing each other, David's eyes grew stronger and softer. And as I watched he became filled with a deep, inner peace. The peace of one who has looked deeply into his heart and soul and discovered a profound truth about himself. The peace of one who has come to know himself as timeless, dimensionless, and eternal—and as not only the source of love but the very essence of love itself.

"I heard Him," David whispered, barely able to talk, but hardly needing to. "I heard Him," he whispered again. "I heard Him."

David had only a short time left to live. Even within that short time, he may not have always remained in the transcendent state of consciousness he experienced that day. But I know he kept the awareness of that state of consciousness and the memory of it, and I know it was a great source of strength for him to call upon. It has also been a source of strength for me, and I'm honored to have been there with David to share it.

SOME PRACTICAL SUGGESTIONS

The purpose of this chapter has been to show the importance of emotional healing and to show the powerful effect it has on the lives of cancer patients and their loved ones. Here are some practical suggestions that can foster this emotional healing at any point in the journey through cancer:

• Remember to get a hard-bound journal, and write about your experiences for at least a few minutes a day. This is as important for spouses and family members as it is for patients.

• Remember, this is your private journal. No one else will see it without your permission. Be honest with yourself. By putting your feelings— all of them—into writing, you will begin to make room for new feelings. You may also find out some surprising things about what your deepest emotions really are. Ask yourself the following questions on a regular basis, and write down your answers without editing or judging them:

1. How do I feel today? What emotions have I experienced in the past twenty-four hours?
2. How do I feel about this cancer? What is it doing to my life?
3. What am I willing to give up because of this cancer?
4. What are the gifts that this cancer can bring to me and my family?
5. What can I do to help myself feel better today?

• Join a support group. It is critical for you to have opportunities to share your feelings with others in a safe and healthy way. Remember that your spouse and family cannot meet all of your emotional needs. It is unfair and unwise to ask them to do so. You can help yourself, and them, by finding other places for support.

• Consider finding a private therapist to talk with on a regular basis. The emotional ups and downs encountered on the journey through cancer may at times call for a professional counselor to help guide you through the most intense periods. If you find you are struggling with depression, anger, despair, fear, guilt, or resentment, it is time to get some help and support. This is equally true for spouses and family members. You can't really help the one you love if you are tied up in emotional knots. Getting help for yourself is one of the greatest gifts you can give to your loved one.

8

LEVEL FIVE: THE NATURE OF MIND

THE GREATEST DISCOVERY OF MY GENERATION IS
THAT A HUMAN BEING CAN ALTER HIS LIFE BY
ALTERING HIS ATTITUDES OF MIND.

—WILLIAM JAMES

Shakespeare wrote, "Nothing is either good or bad, but thinking makes it so." This is the essence of the ideas we'll be discussing in this chapter, and I emphasize that these thoughts must be applied with great care and sensitivity in the journey through cancer. I don't intend to suggest that cancer is caused by "wrong" thoughts, or that it can be cured by thinking "right" ones. And I absolutely don't intend to suggest that getting cancer is "good." However, the *experience* of cancer is always and absolutely a *subjective* one. Recognizing this, we can discuss some important ways in which the journey can be transformed by understanding how our mental processes profoundly affect our experiences in the real world.

THOUGHTS

Although many thousands of thoughts race through your mind during your waking hours, there is surprisingly little variation among them from one day to the next. It is true that what you think about on a fishing trip to Alaska will be different from your thoughts during a meeting at your office, but the vast background of memories, worries, and aspirations changes very slowly over the course of years. From day to day or week to week there may be virtually no change at all. In this sense, our minds are like rivers, streaming with thoughts that flow along preexisting ruts and rivulets.

Despite the sheer numbers of our thoughts, it is a fact of cognitive psychology that we can experience only one of them at a time. A classic demonstration of this involves asking someone *not* to think of the color green. If you really try this, you'll find that your intention *not to think of the color green* overrides your ability to focus elsewhere, and mental images of grass, trees, and dollar bills may crowd your thinking process. Actually, every one of our thoughts pulls on our attention in the same way, but we are generally unaware of this. Our thoughts also move along so quickly that we experience them as a continuous stream, rather than as discrete objects. This process is much like the single frames of film that portray fluid motion when projected in a moving sequence onto a movie screen. Here, each frame is an individual thought; the movie screen is the screen of our awareness; and the movie itself is our perception and experience of "reality."

A diagnosis of cancer has an instant and extremely powerful effect on these characteristics of the thinking process. The consistency that characterized your thoughts from day to day suddenly changes. As the well-worn course of your mental stream abruptly veers off in a new direction, the effect can be profoundly destabilizing. The habitual thought patterns with which you were so comfortable—perhaps even too comfortable—are overridden as the mind tries to orient itself in new and uncharted territory. Moreover, the content of your thoughts often changes from a sequence of vaguely related or completely random entities to a single preoccupation.

In the past, your mind may have made a series of quick mental leaps from wondering where to eat lunch, to thinking about your children, to considering a problem at your job. Now there are just variations on a single theme: "Why did I get cancer? Where can I get the best treatment? I'm terrified…what is going to happen to me?"

Another metaphor for the activity of the mind can be found in the Eastern traditions of meditation. Here the mind is sometimes described as a monkey, jumping incessantly from tree to tree, never stopping except when we are in deep sleep. In normal life, the "monkey mind" jumps from thought to thought, covering a wide range of subjects. But with a diagnosis of cancer the monkey mind can suddenly seem trapped in a forest of ominous and forbidding trees. Wherever it jumps, only dark thoughts are found.

Just as it does in the body, cancer can metastasize in the mind.

Subjectively, the tendency of cancer to monopolize mental content is experienced as *intrusive thought*. In the midst of any activity, a thought related to the illness may suddenly appear, with disruptive effects. Most often these intrusive thoughts are dominated by doubts, judgments, fears, and anxieties, and because they can be so common and so compelling on the journey through cancer, it is important to recognize their effects and bring them under control. Here is an example of how this process works, and how it can be changed:

Mrs. Caldwell was late for her appointment. When I came into the examination room, her eyes were downcast, and I immediately sensed that she was not doing very well.

"Hi, Sarah," I said. "How are you today?"

"Okay, I guess," she said, barely hiding her sadness.

Sarah Caldwell is a fifty-two-year-old woman who had been diagnosed with Stage II breast cancer three months earlier. She had undergone a right modified radical mastectomy and axillary lymph node dissection, and a metastatic tumor was found in four of her lymph nodes. She was now undergoing treatment with adjuvant chemotherapy with the aim of decreasing her chances of relapse.

This is the standard approach, one that tens of thousands of women in America go through every year. Depending on the drugs used, the schedules and doses given, and the individual person, the toxicity from various chemotherapy regimens can vary from virtually none to life-threatening. Mrs. Caldwell was receiving a moderately intense regimen of three drugs that she was tolerating remarkably well; she had not suffered any fatigue, loss of appetite, nausea, vomiting, mouth sores, or fevers of any kind after two cycles. But one major problem had come up—and even though we had talked about it, and she knew it was coming, she hadn't expected it to hit her so hard.

The problem was alopecia—hair loss. This occurs quite dramatically with a number of chemotherapy drugs, including one that Sarah was taking. Over the past few weeks, at first in small strands and then later in clumps, and finally in what seemed to her like an avalanche over a few days, all of her hair had fallen out.

I knew how devastating this could be—and also how devastating the *thought* of it and the *fear* of it could be. I knew women who had avoided chemotherapy, and had very likely shortened their lives, because they were terrified of losing their hair. Some were not able to admit this was the reason they renounced the treatments, and they looked for medical or philosophical reasons that seemed easier to legitimize. But the real reason was the pain, loss of control, and loss of self-esteem they associated with losing their hair. If that wasn't painful enough, they often felt too afraid or ashamed to admit this and discuss it openly with the doctor to whom they had entrusted their lives.

Sarah was usually a cheerful person, who loved to laugh and make light of whatever was happening, but today I could tell she was at a real low point. Together we had faced her diagnosis, surgery, and pathology reports head-on. We had also faced her fears about chemotherapy, and she had found the strength to go forward and successfully complete her first two cycles of treatment with virtually no problems. But the experience of losing her hair was something else altogether. She looked forlorn, stranded, trapped.

"I know this is hard for you," I said. "Why don't you tell me what's going on inside?"

Looking up at me, her eyes suddenly filled with tears and she started sobbing uncontrollably. "Dr. Geffen," she cried, "I can't stand it. Every time I look at myself in the mirror, I feel so ugly. I don't want to look like this. Without any hair, I look just like a man. I feel so ugly...and I feel like I'm going to die."

The depth of her pain was raw and clear; it was heartbreaking to see. But at the same time I was also very proud of her. She was beginning to confront what her illness and the effects of her treatment really meant to her. It took real courage to face this so directly.

"Basically I feel okay about the chemotherapy treatments," she continued. "But I'm horrified every time I look in the mirror and see I'm bald. I just feel so *ugly,* and *I feel like I'm going to die.*" As these thoughts and images reentered her mind, her whole physiology transformed. Within seconds she was crying and sobbing again.

"Sarah," I finally said, "may I ask you a question?"

"Okay."

"How many times a day do you look in a mirror?"

"I don't know," she said, turning away.

"Really, Sarah—how many times a day do you look in a mirror?"

She paused for a long time, fighting the question. Finally, she answered softly, her eyes looking downward, "Well, maybe four times a day."

She then looked at me, and without speaking another word we both knew that the real answer was probably more like forty times a day, or perhaps even 140. But the actual number was unimportant compared to the emotional pain she was experiencing and the effect it could have on her treatment.

"Sarah, do you have any idea what these thoughts might be doing to your energy level and to your ability to heal in this situation? What do you think happens to your heart, your spirit, and even your physical body when you look at yourself in the mirror and have these kind of thoughts over and over again?"

"I don't know," she said.

"Well, maybe we can find out. Are you willing to try?"

"Okay," she answered.

"All right, then," I said. "Now sit up straight, and take a deep breath. I want you to close your eyes and imagine you are at home, standing in front of your mirror, looking at yourself like you normally do."

Sarah closed her eyes, and I watched her face closely. Soon, I could see that, in her thoughts, she was approaching the mirror and the familiar tape was beginning to run: *"I'm so ugly, I'm so ugly, I'm going to die."* Suddenly, she started crying again, literally bent over in pain, suffering exactly as if the whole experience she was imagining was *actually happening.*

"Sarah, look inside your heart and take another deep breath," I said. "Now, focus your awareness for a moment away from your thoughts and into your heart, deep inside of yourself. Take yet another deep breath, and focus again on your heart. As you exhale let the thoughts go and settle even deeper into your heart. Now, let your awareness expand, and observe what you're experiencing."

As her thoughts shifted focus, her crying stopped and she calmed down considerably. But her face still wore a look of great sadness. Finally she opened her eyes. "It's awful, Dr. Geffen," she said. "I feel so hopeless and unlovable. Look at me, I'm so ugly, so *disfigured*. And I feel like I'm going to die."

"Sarah, can you see what these thoughts might be doing to you, and what effect they might have if they continue on like this for weeks and months?"

"Yes," she said, then paused for a long moment. "They might *really* make me die."

This was a moment of genuine revelation for her. She had just witnessed a profound truth about what she was doing to herself with her own thoughts. She had seen how powerful and destructive her thought patterns could be. Even if they did not actually make her die physically, she realized how they were standing firmly in the way of finding inner peace and a deep experience of healing.

I allowed some time to pass for the full impact of what she had discovered to sink into her awareness. Then I gently said, "Sarah, may I ask you another question now?"

"Okay," she said.

"Did you ever think of how extraordinary it is that you love yourself enough, and you want to live enough, that you would go through all of this in order to stay alive? That you would face even your worst fears in order to save your life?"

The look on her face in the next few moments was precious beyond words. In an instant her mind and heart and body had suddenly begun to discover an entirely new meaning in everything she had been going through. It was as if some dark gray cloud in the sky of her mind was parting, floating away, and rays of sunlight were beginning to stream through, tentatively at first but then stronger and stronger.

"Did you ever think," I continued, "that going through all of this is a statement not only of how strong and courageous you are, but of how *beautiful* you are?"

Sarah was now sitting up much straighter. Spontaneously, her breathing had become deeper and more confident. I asked her if she was willing to take this understanding one step further. When she answered yes, I asked her to stay still for a moment. Then I went out of the room and asked one of our staff members for a mirror.

Back in the examination room, I asked Sarah to hold the mirror in front of her and to look directly into it.

This was difficult for her to do, and she kept looking away. She wanted to look at anything other than the mirror. I gently encouraged her to take this important step, but she just couldn't do it.

"I know it's scary," I said, "but I want to help you anchor in this new meaning that you have for how you look. I'd also like to help you feel differently about mirrors. Are you willing to do this?"

Slowly, very slowly, she answered, "Well…okay." But she was still not able to look at herself in the mirror.

So I asked her again to close her eyes. "Sarah, I want you to remember now where you were just a few moments ago. Remember feeling your strength and courage. Remember feeling how much you love yourself, so much, in fact, that you are willing to fight hard to stay alive. Can you feel this now, and appreciate how extraordinary it is? Allow yourself the pleasure of feeling how much you really do love yourself, and how courageous and beautiful you are."

I watched as a new wave of love and appreciation for herself started to flow through her body. Something so life-giving was beautiful to see. After a while she was smiling again and opened her eyes.

"Okay, Sarah, I want you to look at yourself in the mirror now. Are you ready?"

This was still a bit scary for her, but after a few additional moments of hesitation, she broke through and jumped right in. Staring at her own sweet, round face and completely bald head in the mirror, she sat there, smiling away.

"Now," I said, "I'd like you to repeat the following words after me. *'Sarah, I love you…'*"

Still staring at herself in the mirror, Sarah again hesitated for a moment. Then, speaking softly to herself, she slowly repeated my words. After she finished, I continued on.

"And I love you so much that I'm willing to fight hard to keep you alive…

"I'm not going to let anything stop you…

"'I'm willing to go through surgery, and chemotherapy, and a lot of pain and inconvenience for you...

"'And I'm even willing to lose all of my hair, if that's what it takes, because I love you so much, and I'm totally committed to you.'"

As she repeated these words, looking directly at herself in the mirror, her face became soft and radiant. Then we sat quietly together as she took a few minutes to absorb and appreciate the full impact of what she had just accomplished, and how far she had come. In this silence her eyes again filled with tears, but this time they were not bitter tears. They were the sweet, nurturing tears that cleanse, heal, and uplift the human heart and spirit.

"Do you feel ugly now?" I asked.

"No," she replied, looking at herself once again in the mirror. "I feel beautiful." Now it seemed that she could barely stop looking at herself in the mirror, smiling, her eyes sparkling in love.

"I feel so beautiful," Sarah said again, then paused before saying, "and I *know* that I'm going to live."

BELIEFS

We've just seen a clear example of how thoughts can have a life of their own, particularly under the stressful conditions encountered in the diagnosis and treatment of cancer. Thoughts are almost always involuntary. In the form of fears, doubts, or apprehensions, they can appear and disappear without any conscious intention on our part. Beliefs also usually arise without our conscious intention or consent, but they involve a higher level of commitment than our thoughts. They are, quite simply, thoughts we have elevated to the level of truth.

For example, we may randomly and momentarily think about the dangers of flying before we board a commercial airline, but we confidently *believe* that we will arrive at our destination safely. Similarly, random thoughts about cancer may go in many different and even contradictory directions over the course of a day. But *beliefs* about cancer are much more deeply ingrained and slower to change. The remarkable thing about these beliefs is that they will influence every aspect of your experience of cancer in a dramatic way. They will also influence virtually all of the decisions about the course of treatment you choose. And thus, they may—in a very real way—affect your ultimate outcome as well.

The hallmark features of our beliefs include how unconscious they are, how pervasive they are, and how precious we hold and regard them. The truth is, we have unconscious beliefs about *everything*, and these act like invisible filters through which we sift everything that occurs in the "outer world." These beliefs are not intrinsically bad; in fact, we could not function without them. But they can become deadly in the face of cancer—unless we are willing to see what they are and consciously choose whether or not they are grounded in fact or fear. One of the saddest commentaries on the human condition is that human beings will kill others or even themselves because of their most deeply held beliefs. I have seen this many times in people who are struggling between the direct, practical realities of their cancer and the conviction of some of their most deeply held and cherished beliefs.

Despite the attachment that exists between people and their beliefs, most of us are largely unaware of how our beliefs developed or how we might benefit if they were changed. Beliefs most often originate in childhood from the statements or actions of individuals we regarded as authority figures. Parents are by far the most important. If your parents told you over and over again that "you can't trust anyone," and scolded you whenever you betrayed this, this very likely became an unconscious belief that will have an effect on your relationships with people throughout your life.

You might think, "Oh, I understand this, and it doesn't affect me anymore," and that may be true to a great extent, especially in normal daily activities. But if you or your spouse is suddenly diagnosed with cancer, and you suddenly feel that your life may be threatened, this deeply seated unconscious belief may suddenly be activated and influence how you interact with everyone—including your spouse or the doctors who are trying to help you. This may be one reason why some people need three, four, or even five "second opinions" before they are willing to accept a physician's recommendations and care.

Human beings have unconscious beliefs about everything, and these influence both our decisions and our experiences of the actions that result from them. I have found that it is extremely important and helpful for people dealing with cancer to take some time out toward the beginning of treatment and explore what some of their beliefs are about matters that will have a great impact on what comes next.

In dealing with patients' beliefs about cancer and cancer treatment, I've found that it's much more useful to ask questions than to make directive statements. Putting questions and answers in written form can be especially illuminating. The concentration demanded by writing allows a different and more objective perspective on beliefs to appear.

I have developed a series of questions for patients and family members to explore and answer. You are encouraged to do this in private, and you don't have to share the results with anyone if you don't want to. But it is helpful to see some of the beliefs you hold, usually unconsciously, so you can decide if you want to change some of them. Very often people discover that they have conflicting beliefs. Discovering this can be very useful and often helps reveal why some decisions seem so much harder to make than others. Here are those questions:

1. What are your beliefs about cancer?
(For example: *Cancer is a deadly process. Cancer is curable. Cancer will wreck my life. Cancer will be a challenge, but it won't destroy me.*)

_____

_____

_____

_____

_____

2. What are your beliefs about doctors?
(For example: *Doctors are knowledgeable, but uncaring. Doctors are knowledgeable, and some of them do care. Doctors are greedy. Doctors are untrustworthy. Doctors are trustworthy. Doctors don't really tell you the truth.*)

_____

_____

_____
_____
_____

3. What are your beliefs about why you got cancer?

(For example: *I got cancer because I smoked cigarettes. Because I ate bad food for many years of my life. Because I lived near a toxic manufacturing plant as a child. Because I lived near power lines for ten years. Because I inherited bad genes from my mother or father. Because I am being tested by God. Because I am being punished by God.*)

_____
_____
_____
_____
_____

4. What are your beliefs about chemotherapy (or radiation, or surgery)?

(For example: *Chemotherapy will save my life. Chemotherapy will not save my life, but will help me live longer. Chemotherapy is poison. Chemotherapy will destroy my immune system. Chemotherapy will make me sick. Chemotherapy is a great gift. Chemotherapy will help me greatly.*)

_____
_____
_____
_____
_____

5. What are your beliefs and expectations about what will happen to you?

(For example: *I will probably die. I may suffer for a while, but I will probably be okay. I don't really know what will happen to me.*)

_____

_____

_____

_____

6. What are your beliefs about God?

(For example: *I don't believe there is a God. I believe that God is nature. I believe there is a supreme being called God who is kind and good. I believe that God is all loving. I believe that God punishes us for our sins.*)

_____

_____

_____

_____

7. What are your beliefs about spirituality?

(For example: *I believe there is a spiritual dimension to life that is real. Spirituality is important to me. I don't believe there is a spiritual dimension to life; what you see is all there is. Spirituality is not important.*)

_____

_____

_____

_____

8. What are your beliefs about death and life after death?
(For example: *I believe that life ends when you die, and that nothing exists beyond death. I believe that we all have a soul that lives on after the body, but I don't know what happens to it after death. I believe in heaven and hell, and that you will be judged and sent to one place or the other. I believe in reincarnation.*)

_____

_____

_____

_____

Here is a story that illustrates how someone's unconscious beliefs about a particular drug greatly influenced her decision whether to have more treatment for breast cancer:

Joyce Holt is a forty-three-year-old registered nurse with extensive medical experience. When she was diagnosed with Stage II breast cancer she suddenly found herself transformed from a caregiver to a patient. After her initial surgery Mrs. Holt was faced with important decisions about adjuvant treatment. She had consultations at several leading cancer centers around the country, and all of them strongly recommended four cycles of chemotherapy with Adriamycin and Cytoxan to be given over twelve weeks, followed by five years of oral hormone therapy with the estrogen-blocking drug tamoxifen. Mrs. Holt readily agreed to the four cycles of chemotherapy, but she felt highly resistant to taking tamoxifen.

My intention is not to argue the merits of tamoxifen. However, it is important to note that tamoxifen is a drug that has been tested successfully in many thousands of women over several decades, and its risks and benefits have been clearly defined. The drug is associated with relatively small but real risks of blood clots, uterine cancer, hot flashes, weight gain, and other potential side effects. But these side effects are balanced with very real and substantial benefits in terms of proven reduction in recurrence of breast cancer, decreased deaths from heart disease, and decreased morbidity from osteoporosis, another potentially life-threatening disease in women.

Every year, thousands of women face the decision of whether to take tamoxifen. The numbers will soon be even higher, because tamoxifen was approved in 1998 as a drug to *prevent* breast cancer in women who are at high risk of developing the disease. Many women readily agree to the recommendation to take tamoxifen because of its measurable, documented, and unmistakably significant benefits—which, in the vast majority of cases, far outweigh its potential risks.

Many other women, however, struggle deeply with the decision. Why? It is usually not because they are unaware of the data or statistics, which clearly spell out the potential benefits of the drug. Rather, when a patient struggles with a decision like this it is because of her *beliefs* about what taking the drug will really *mean* in her life.

Mrs. Holt was such a patient. A highly intelligent, highly educated professional nurse, she was fully conversant with all of the arguments about tamoxifen's risks and benefits. Yet, even though she had readily agreed to undergo initial treatment with Adriamycin and Cytoxan—drugs which in many ways are much more "toxic" than tamoxifen—she felt uncomfortable at the prospect of taking tamoxifen. The more strongly it was recommended by various physicians, the more resistant she became.

When I spoke with Mrs. Holt about this, she was uncharacteristically emotional and defensive about her feelings. "I just don't want to take it," she said emphatically. "I know about the data and all that, and I know it might be a mistake. But I just don't want to do it."

I quickly realized that something deeper was going on here. There was no question in my mind that this otherwise calm and clear-headed woman was having an emotional reaction to conscious—or unconscious—fears and beliefs. I also realized that trying to "talk her into" taking tamoxifen—regardless of how strongly I felt it would be good for her—was doomed to failure because she was not approaching this particular decision from a rational place. She had already made up her mind. Furthermore, I was sure that if I pushed her to take tamoxifen I would destroy the trust and rapport we had carefully and tenderly built in our relationship over the prior months of treatment. If I tried to influence her decision by intimidating her, or filling her mind with more fear—specifically with ominous references to how her cancer could "come back" if she didn't take tamoxifen—I knew I would drive a wedge between us and make it harder for her to trust and count on me.

Whether Mrs. Holt's fears and beliefs about tamoxifen were accurate was not the point. This was someone I cared about, and I could see she was in pain. She was also making a decision that I honestly believed was not in her best interests. I realized, though, that she was a bright and intelligent woman who was capable of making the best choice for herself *if* she really had *all* the information she needed. Although she had facts and figures about the risks and benefits of tamoxifen, she didn't have the information *about her own conscious or unconscious fears and beliefs* that were so obviously influencing her decision. What was ultimately important to me was that she make her decision, whatever that might be, from a place of real strength, confidence, knowledge, and wisdom—rather than from fear, uncertainty, and potentially inaccurate and disempowering beliefs.

I asked Mrs. Holt if she would be interested in exploring exactly what was going on inside her mind and heart, either consciously or unconsciously, that was so strongly influencing her decision to refuse tamoxifen. I reassured her that I would accept whatever decision she chose, and not try to pressure her. However, I did want to help her find real clarity and peace of mind about her decision. After she felt reassured, she agreed.

I then asked Mrs. Holt to write down, in a general way, her principal beliefs about tamoxifen. These were her responses:

My beliefs about tamoxifen are . . .
1. It has many side effects.
2. It is an unnatural and unhealthy substance.
3. It will make me have hot flashes.
4. It will decrease my sex drive.
5. It will increase my risk of uterine cancer.
6. It will disrupt the hormonal equilibrium of my body, which I believe goes against the laws of nature and is not good for me.

Mrs. Holt and I then discussed her beliefs in detail. I didn't do so with the intention of arguing with her or convincing her she was wrong, or right. What she had written, after all, was certainly understandable from her perspective. I simply asked her how and why she believed these particular things about tamoxifen, how certain she felt that she would experience the side effects she listed, and *why*. In general, tamoxifen is a drug with relatively low toxicity. As a medical professional, Mrs. Holt was aware of that. But beliefs are not necessarily determined by known facts, and just by asking her questions in a nonjudgmental way she acknowledged that she really wasn't *sure* she would experience every one of the side effects she listed, but she was *afraid* she would. Even though she also knew that she could stop taking tamoxifen *at any time* if she did experience any of the unwanted side effects, she was still adamant about not even trying it.

Without contradicting what Mrs. Holt said or had written, I asked her to think for a few moments and list some of her thoughts about what it might cost her to hold on to her particular beliefs about tamoxifen, particularly if it meant that she would ultimately decide not to take it as prescribed. This was not asserting that she was wrong, but simply focusing on the results her beliefs could bring about. It was a matter of asking her a question and letting her provide the answers.

What could holding on to my beliefs about tamoxifen **cost** *me?*
1. A possible recurrence.
2. A lot of grief as a result of a recurrence.
3. Irreplaceable time with my husband.
4. Increased risk of heart disease and osteoporosis.
5. It could cost me my life, if I were to have a recurrence.

Finally, I asked Mrs. Holt to write down what she could possibly gain from taking tamoxifen.

What could I possibly **gain** *by taking tamoxifen?*
1. I could improve my chances of not having a recurrence and living a long and healthy life.
2. I could significantly improve my chances of avoiding heart disease and osteoporosis.

3. I could gain the knowledge that I was getting the benefit of everything medical science has to offer me right now.
4. I could gain the benefit of making my husband feel reassured.

It is fascinating to realize the extent to which Mrs. Holt's responses
go directly to the heart of her personal hopes and fears. These are concerns that would never have come up if I had simply presented the statistics about adjuvant therapy with tamoxifen. If I had said, "Here are the
numbers, now you decide," her core issues would have remained unac-
knowledged and unresolved—and the deepest possible healing would
not have taken place, regardless of whether she took tamoxifen.

Once Mrs. Holt's negative fears and beliefs were clearly revealed to
herself, and their possible costs were weighed against the possible benefits of treatment, it was easy for her to make the prudent decision of
going ahead with the therapy. While I do believe that this was the wisest
choice for her, the *way* she made her decision was just as important to
me, as was the sense of clarity and empowerment she had afterward. It
was now truly *her choice,* not mine or anyone else's. Furthermore, since
her mind and her heart were now aligned with the decision, I felt certain
that she would have no unnecessary toxicities that can arise when treatment choices are made from fear-based, unconscious beliefs, or when
they are made with doubts and ambivalence. I also felt certain that she
would now get the most benefit possible from her treatment, because she
had come to the decision on her own, with real understanding and
insight about what was most important to her.

MEANINGS

If beliefs are the "truths" we attach to ideas and experiences in the real
world, meanings are the *significance* we give to those ideas and experiences. The mind assigns meaning to virtually everything it focuses upon,
and the degree of significance can range from the unimportant and triv-
ial to the highly spiritual and profound. In fact, whenever *anything* happens within our awareness, our mind assigns it a meaning. Just as with
our thoughts and beliefs, this process is usually unconscious and instan-
taneous. To a greater degree than most people ever suspect, the meaning

we assign to events fundamentally affects our entire experience of life in that moment.

If your boss calls you unexpectedly one day, the meaning you consciously or unconsciously assign to the call determines whether you are filled with fear, curiosity, elation, or dread. If you think the call means you are about to be fired, you might feel fear and tension. But if you think you are about to be given a raise, you might feel elation. And if you have no idea what the call "means," your mind will start searching for a meaning. *"What is this call about? Did I do something wrong?"*

Similarly, if your spouse does not show up to meet you at the time you agreed upon, the *meaning* you give to his or her absence will determine how you feel. If your mind thinks the reason your spouse is late is because *"he was in a car accident and he was hurt,"* you will have one kind of experience internally. On the other hand, if your mind says something like, *"She is always late. I can never count on her to keep her word. She doesn't respect me!"* you will have an entirely different experience.

The point here is that in both of these situations, *as with every situation that we can or will ever experience in life,* it is not the event that determines our experience, but the *meaning* and *significance* we give it. I realize this is a radical assertion, but there is no question in my mind that it is true—and it is especially true when dealing with cancer. I have seen over and over again how the *meaning* cancer patients give to their illness can dramatically affect how they respond to diagnosis, choose treatment, and deal with possible side effects. What is often overlooked in this process is how these meanings can have very negative—as well as positive—effects.

Most people are comfortable with the meaning they ascribe to their situation in life, but others may find themselves chronically unhappy or unable to change habitual self-sabotaging patterns in their lives. Often some personal conviction—deeply held but incompletely understood—stops them from moving forward. For a physician, helping patients to identify and understand the meanings they find in illnesses should be an important element of the treatment process.

The contrasting experiences of two patients with virtually identical diagnoses provides a dramatic illustration of this. But before recounting the story, let me pause to make an important observation. Again and again in my work as an oncologist I've seen the importance of God and religion in the lives of a large percentage of patients. Although religion may not play a major role in everyone's life, it is extremely important to a great many people in our society. During a crisis like cancer it often, and understandably, becomes even more important. The frequency with which God is mentioned in this book is not an attempt to proselytize, judge, or even comment upon the value or significance of religion. Nor is it necessarily a reflection of my own personal beliefs. It is simply a reflection of what oncologists often encounter in dealing with real patients in the real world.

At the age of fifty-four, Ken Mitchell was found to have extensive lung and liver metastases of a high-grade malignant melanoma. He was a devoted family man, with a profound religious faith. His diagnosis plunged him into a deep depression, and nothing seemed to help him feel better emotionally. Despite everyone's attempt to reach out to him he remained angry, bitter, and resentful. After many soul-searching conversations, I asked Mr. Mitchell if he would tell me his thoughts about the meaning of his illness and why he believed he got cancer. "I'm a sinner, Dr. Geffen," he confided in me. "God gave me this illness to punish me for my sins."

Michael Hart, also fifty-four, was diagnosed with the same cancer as Mr. Mitchell. He too was very devoted to his family and to his religion. After his diagnosis, Mr. Hart did not sink into despair. Instead, he focused even more intently than before on the people in his life he cared most about. He refused to feel sorry for himself or to become depressed, and never sank into self-pity or resentment. In the midst of his overwhelmingly challenging situation, he was calm, cheerful, and optimistic—and everyone who met him was uplifted simply by being in his presence. I asked him how he did it, and what his thoughts were about the meaning of his illness, and why he believed he got cancer.

"I don't really know why I got cancer, Doc," he explained. "But I do know this—this experience is making me a better, stronger person. And it is bringing me closer to my Creator, to myself, and to the people I love—closer than I could have ever imagined. So, no matter what happens, it's okay. I know I've been given this challenge for a purpose that can and will serve me and those I love. As a matter of fact, how are you doing, Doc? Don't forget, I'm praying for *you* every single day."

What was the difference between Mr. Mitchell and Mr. Hart? Their medical situations were as similar as the importance of family and religion in their lives. But because of the different *meaning* they gave to their illnesses, they were living in two completely different worlds. This had a direct bearing on their experiences during treatment and strongly influenced everyone around them as well.

These distinctions are merely a glimpse of the understanding and clarity that this level of the program gives to patients and family members. My goal is to help patients and family members discover and explore the beliefs, values, and meanings they would consciously choose to have at this most critical time in their lives—beliefs, values, and meanings that are empowering, uplifting, and health-promoting, rather than the unconscious beliefs, values, and meanings that they may carry with them from their past, which may not be supporting them at all.

Focus

Another important component of the activity of our mind can contribute significantly to how we feel and respond to any experience, including the experience of cancer. I refer to this component as *focus*. Our experience of events is not only influenced by our thoughts, beliefs, and ascribed meanings but by *what we focus on*. This is a basic tenet of biofeedback, which trains people how to consciously redirect their focus away from unpleasant thoughts or emotions and toward pleasant and relaxing ones. By changing your focus, you can change how you feel.

There are many examples of this, and the effects can be both positive and negative. For example, ignoring the warning signs of cancer by focusing on something else can lead to a crucial delay in diagnosis. Conversely, focusing only on possible adverse side effects of cancer treatment can make the experience significantly more difficult and actually leads some people to forgo potentially life-saving therapies.

There is no question that patients who are able to shift their focus in positive ways not only have a less stressful experience with challenges like cancer but also often have better outcomes. In fact, an area where this is repeatedly seen in medicine involves people with strong religious faith. Without attempting to answer the question of whether people are indeed able to draw upon a higher power, or the extent to which a strong spiritual or religious faith may make a difference in a particular patient's clinical course, it is very clear that it allows many patients to radically change their focus in the face of great, or even overwhelming, challenges. The following story illustrates how clear and how powerful this can be when it occurs.

Jack Montgomery was a delightful seventy-eight-year-old gentleman from Georgia who had been admitted to the hospital with fever, a productive cough, and abdominal pain of several days duration. CT scans of his chest and abdomen were highly suggestive of a primary lung cancer, with extensive liver metastases. I was called to see him for consultation on a Saturday, as he and his family awaited the results of a liver biopsy to determine the nature of his apparent malignancy.

For fifty years Mr. Montgomery had worked as a carpenter and also as a gardener. He loved to grow his own food, and his face and skin were thickened and engraved with lines that looked like tire treads from spending so many years in the hot Georgia sun. He was most proud when his son and daughter grew up, got married, and had children, whom he loved dearly. Like most men of his time, Mr. Montgomery smoked cigarettes. In fact, he had smoked at least one or two packs of cigarettes a day for nearly fifty years.

As we got to know each other, Mr. Montgomery tried to put up a brave face in light of his impending diagnosis. At moments, however, he would let down enough to allow me to see the intense fear and sadness in his heart as he thought about the idea of having cancer and possibly dying. Most of all, he was overwhelmed with grief at the thought of leaving his beloved family.

When I arrived at the hospital the following Monday morning, I went immediately to the pathology department and reviewed Mr. Montgomery's slides. The diagnosis of extensive-stage small-cell carcinoma of the lung was unequivocal. With a heavy heart, I made my way up to Mr.

Montgomery's room, wishing there was a way to avoid giving him and his family the information for which they were waiting.

As I entered Mr. Montgomery's room, I found his family surrounding his bed. There were his wife, his son and daughter, his son-in-law and daughter-in-law, and his brother. We greeted one another and made small talk for a few minutes, trying to ease the obvious fear and tension in the air. Finally, I could delay the discussion no further.

"Mr. Montgomery," I began, "I have some results of your liver biopsy now, if you would like to discuss them."

I looked at him lying in bed and waited for his acknowledgment before going further. Mr. Montgomery closed his eyes, as if bracing himself, and gently nodded his head. He then opened his eyes again and looked at me.

"Unfortunately," I continued, as gently as I could, "the biopsy has confirmed that the mass in your lung is a lung cancer, and it has spread into your liver."

Silence came over the room as the family tried to absorb this. I searched for something further to say. If I told Mr. Montgomery his disease was incurable, all hope would have been destroyed in a heartbeat. He might have felt deeply abandoned, and any belief in the possibility of meaningful survival, let alone unexpected cures, would be greatly diminished in his mind and heart. On the other hand, it is cruel and unfair to overstate what one can reasonably expect to achieve with conventional medicine. There is a fine line between "telling the truth" and not destroying a patient's hope and spirit.

Facing many such moments over the years, I have developed a personal style that seems to work well for both my patients and myself. I always try to find something positive and hopeful to say about the situation, no matter how grim it may be. In this case, the specific subtype of his lung cancer gave me a very real potential opening.

"Mr. Montgomery," I said, "the kind of lung cancer that you have is the small-cell type. This type tends to be readily treatable. We can definitely treat you with chemotherapy, and it is also very possible that chemotherapy will be of benefit, perhaps even significant benefit."

"But is it curable, Dr. Geffen? Can you cure me?"

"Mr. Montgomery," I said, "I have to tell you that it is very, very diffi-cult to cure this kind of lung cancer with the treatments that are available right now. I'm not saying it *can't* be cured, because there is always a great mystery in what ultimately happens to any of us in life. And my own conviction and experience in these kinds of situations is that, in truth, *anything* can happen, including being cured, even when that doesn't seem likely or possible. But it is also important for you to understand that this kind of disease is usually extremely difficult, if not impossible, to cure, particularly when it has already spread so extensively. Nonetheless, we can definitely treat it, if you wish, and try to get it under control at least for a while. And if the treatments are successful, then it will help you feel a lot better. And it may help you live longer, too."

After a long silence, Mrs. Montgomery finally spoke. She was sitting in a chair in the corner of the room, literally trembling, fighting back tears.

"Dr. Geffen," she asked, "how long are we talking about if my hus-band takes chemotherapy? And how long will he live if he doesn't take chemotherapy?"

For an oncologist, these are some of the most difficult questions that can be asked by terrified patients and family members. They are also some of the most common. Typically, the physician responds by citing published survival statistics. For a man like Mr. Montgomery, the median survival is several months, which might or might not be pro-longed by treatment. However, blurting out numbers in a situation like this is, I believe, insensitive and cruel. I also believe it is misleading. Every human being is absolutely unique, and no one can predict with any certainty how long any one of us is going to live. Every oncologist has seen patients with advanced cancer who died much sooner than anyone expected. And there are also many patients who lived far, far longer than the "median survival statistics" would predict.

Patients and family members are looking for a specific time frame in this situation. They want some certainty about what to expect. Unfortu-nately, the sense of certainty that patients get when they are told, "You have three to six months to live," often turns out to be completely wrong. Or it becomes a self-fulfilling prophecy.

When I try to answer these questions without giving specific num-bers, many times patients feel somewhat frustrated. I believe the answer

I commonly give is much gentler to their hearts, even if their minds are not entirely satisfied.

"Well, Mrs. Montgomery," I began, "the question that you are asking me is very reasonable, very real, and very understandable. I am asked that question almost every day by patients and their families. Unfortunately, it is very difficult to answer with any certainty. There are various published statistics that suggest what the average survival of patients in this kind of situation is, but I hesitate to draw on those statistics or give them too much credence. Your husband is not a statistic. He is a unique, very special and precious individual and no one can truly predict his destiny in this situation. Some lung cancer patients live only a few weeks, with or without chemotherapy. Others, particularly those who have successful chemotherapy treatment, can live for many, many months. Occasionally, some will live even longer still. It's very difficult to predict in any individual case."

I then paused once again as this painful but honest information was slowly assimilated by Mr. Montgomery and his family.

After some time, Mr. Montgomery looked up at me from his bed and said, "Well, Dr. Geffen, what should I do?"

This is yet another difficult question. In the field of oncology, in many situations the best option for a given patient is straightforward. Many other times, however, it is not clear at all, and this was the case in Mr. Montgomery's situation. His type of malignancy can be sensitive to chemotherapy, and I have seen extraordinary responses on many occasions, even in elderly patients with advanced disease. If he tolerated chemotherapy well, and if his tumor was responsive, he might indeed gain a great deal from having treatment. On the other hand, Mr. Montgomery was elderly, not in the best overall shape, and furthermore, had *very advanced* cancer. His liver function was already showing signs of compromise. He also had severe underlying emphysema and a weak heart as well. Treating patients with chemotherapy in these kinds of circumstances is much harder and more dangerous. Although Mr. Montgomery was looking to me for guidance, it was difficult to know what was best for him.

"Mr. Montgomery," I began, "let me tell you how other people in your situation have approached this. Some patients feel that if there is some reasonable hope of benefit from treatment, they want to go ahead with it. Those patients understand that chemotherapy can be difficult at times, even when the patient is young, and at your age it can be even harder. Nevertheless, some patients are willing to accept this, because they want to do everything they can to fight and prolong their lives. They are simply not ready to let go.

"Other people take a different approach. These are patients who say, 'Well, regardless of my age, I feel that I've lived a good life. If this chemotherapy is not going to cure me then I'm not sure I want to spend the time I have left on this earth undergoing treatment, running back and forth to the doctor's office and spending time away from my family.' Those patients feel that they are ready to think about letting go and not going through the struggle of battling cancer.

"I want to emphasize to you, Mr. Montgomery, that in my mind either one of these approaches is perfectly reasonable and acceptable. If you want to have treatment and if you want to fight, then I am ready to roll up my sleeves and fight with you. On the other hand, if you feel that you're not up for that kind of struggle at this point, then that too is reasonable. Ultimately, this is a personal choice that you and your family will want to make together."

We then had a detailed conversation about the range of chemotherapy treatments that might be appropriate for Mr. Montgomery, covering the expected benefits as well as the possible side effects. When we had gone over all these issues, there seemed to be nothing left to say. Mr. Montgomery and his family were facing one of the most difficult decisions of their lives. Without anyone saying so directly, it was clear from the tone and direction of their questions that different family members felt very differently—but very strongly—about the best way to proceed.

Then, something extraordinary happened. Mr. Montgomery reached out and asked if he could take my hand in his. He grasped my hand tightly and held it to his chest. Closing his eyes, Mr. Montgomery began to speak in his thick Georgian drawl. He began to pray.

"Lord Jesus, I'm lying here in this moment and calling out to you for help and guidance. Lord Jesus, I don't know which way to go. I pray for your guidance.

"But Lord," Mr. Montgomery continued, "before I ask you for your help, I want to praise you and honor you and thank you from the depths of my heart for all of your blessings in my life. Lord, I *thank you* for all you have given to me and my family for so many years. I *thank you* and *praise you* for your love and your guidance and protection. Thank you for guiding us, and for lifting us up. Lord, we love you and honor you and thank you. *Thank you*, Jesus. Thank you, thank you."

As Mr. Montgomery prayed, tears started welling up in my eyes, and a surge of love filled my heart like a big wave. I was afraid that this wave would rise and rise and spill over, and I would start weeping, because I was so moved by his pure, raw, and absolutely breathtaking declaration of love and gratitude to God.

I glanced around the room and saw everyone standing silently, their hands clasped together. Everyone's head was bowed in reverent prayer, and I realized that—in truth—church, or temple, or whatever you want to call it, is created *instantly* when human beings simply turn their hearts and minds toward God. There, at 9:03 A.M. on a Monday morning in room 468 of Indian River Memorial Hospital, we were all in a sacred space. And Jack Montgomery's prayer had brought us there.

"Lord," he went on, "now I need your help. I am facing a very difficult decision, Lord. It's the hardest one I've ever faced in my life, and I don't know which way to go. Lord, I want you to guide me and guide my family so we can know which road to take. Lord, please above all give your blessings to my family. And Lord, please bless this doctor who also loves you.

"Lord, guide me and show me what is your will. If it's my time to leave this earth, then so be it. Then take me, Lord. Forgive me for my sins and my trespasses and take me home to you. If you want me to fight this disease, then show me how, Lord, and give me the strength and courage to fight. Whatever you wish, Lord, that is the wish of my heart. I want nothing else. Please love and bless my beloved family, Lord. In Jesus' name we honor and praise you. Thank you. Amen."

During his prayer, which was so profound and heartfelt, the space in the room had become completely transformed. The presence of love and grace filled every heart and every corner of that room. The fear and discord had been instantly transformed into unity and gratitude. The members of

Mr. Montgomery's family were holding each other, blowing their noses, and offering each other Kleenex. In those few short moments the unmistakable love, courage, and faith of this man and his family were established beyond question.

It was extraordinary to see how powerfully and elegantly Mr. Montgomery had responded to hearing from his physician that he had a very advanced form of lung cancer that had spread into his liver and was very difficult, if not impossible, to cure. Yet Mr. Montgomery completely transformed the fear and distress of this moment by simply *shifting his focus,* turning to his spiritual faith. He believed he would be guided by a higher power, and he put his focus there. In doing so, he transformed not only his own experience but *everyone else's as well.* His prayer and the power of his faith and focus created an absolutely sublime and healing experience for everyone in the room. I only wished that every human being could face terrifying circumstances with such calm, clear, equanimity and joy in one's heart. I also believed that through this process, Mr. Montgomery had opened himself and his family to the possibility of a deeper healing of the mind, heart, and spirit—as well as the body—of everyone involved.

I reached down and gave Mr. Montgomery a big hug. He grabbed me tightly, as if we had known each other forever. "Thank you, Doctor," he said. "I would like to ask if I can have a day to think about everything and make my decision."

"Of course. Please take all the time you need."

As I was preparing to leave, I noticed how much I wanted to stay in the room. It was an amazing realization. Here I was, the doctor of this beautiful man who had just been diagnosed with metastatic lung cancer, and *I* felt healed by his prayers. How fortunate I am, I thought to myself, to have had this experience this morning. I also thought to myself how blessed this man and his family were to have such a clear and strong spiritual faith. I felt I couldn't leave without acknowledging at least some of this, in some way.

"Mr. Montgomery," I said, "I want you to know how moved and grateful I am to have had this experience with you this morning. I wish that so many other of my patients could have the experience that we've just had. I feel deeply honored to know you, and thank you for including me in your prayers."

With tears still running down her cheeks, Mrs. Montgomery then looked at me and said, "Dr. Geffen, our faith has always guided and sustained us, and it always will. It is the most precious thing we have."

Finally, I pulled myself away from the extraordinary presence of love surrounding this family and, holding back tears of my own, went out in the hall and took a few deep breaths before moving on in my rounds.

My next patient that morning was in many ways strikingly similar, yet radically different. Mr. Bruce was a seventy-six-year-old man who had been undergoing treatment for a chronic blood disorder, which had recently transformed into full-blown acute leukemia.

Both Mr. Bruce and his wife were bitter, angry, and depressed, and visiting with them was always a challenge. Over the six months I had known them, I had tried to engage Mr. and Mrs. Bruce on a personal and empathetic level, but to no avail. I had always been rebuffed with more questions about Mr. Bruce's blood counts, a journal article Mrs. Bruce had found, or possible new treatments.

Before I was even through the door, Mrs. Bruce was demanding to know her husband's morning white blood cell count, whether his hemoglobin had shifted today, and what his platelet count was. She was consistently dissatisfied with the nursing care, demanding that Mr. Bruce be turned more frequently or that his vital signs not be taken so often. The food was always either too hot or too cold, too mushy or too firm, and she couldn't understand why in the world her husband should have to go through any of this. She also demanded that I not fully disclose how dreadful his prognosis truly was. She kept repeating that he would not be able to handle the truth. "I know him better than all of you," she said over and over. "I know that he can't handle it. He'll start crying, and crying…"

I calmly looked at her and said gently, "Mrs. Bruce, what's so wrong and terrible about the possibility that your husband might cry if he learns that he has leukemia, and that he might be dying?"

A long pregnant pause followed, and then the truth was revealed. With tears welling up in her own eyes, she said, "I just can't stand to see him cry."

In her resistance to her own pain and grief, Mrs. Bruce was making herself, her husband, and every one around them miserable. The contrast with Mr. Montgomery's room, only a few yards away, was too clear to ignore. Here were two men in their late seventies, both diagnosed with a serious advanced malignancy, and their *focus* completely determined their experience. How I wished that Mrs. Bruce could have the courage, and the willingness, to allow her own pain and heartbreak to come out. How I wish that she could feel the grace and blessing that Mrs. Montgomery and her family had experienced through the prayers of Mr. Montgomery, as he surrendered and asked for guidance from a higher power, and listened with humility and serenity to whatever answer he would hear in his heart. With this awareness, I sent as much love and compassion as I could to Mrs. Bruce and her beloved husband. For the hundredth time we went over all of the available options and again acknowledged how limited they were.

As I left Mr. Bruce's room and moved on in my rounds, I understood once again how profoundly our thoughts and beliefs, the meanings we give to events, and the focus we bring to them affects every aspect of our lives. Blindly spending millions of dollars on many aspects of cancer treatment seems absurd when a simple act of faith and trust can alleviate so much pain and suffering. I then prayed silently in my own heart for the strength and courage to continue in this effort to realize a vision of medicine that honors and cares not only for the body, but for the mind, heart, and spirit as well.

9

LEVEL SIX:
LIFE ASSESSMENT

> YOU MUST GIVE BIRTH TO YOUR IMAGES.
> THEY ARE THE FUTURE WAITING TO BE BORN.
> —RAINER MARIA RILKE

evel Six of this program is an invitation to explore, discover, understand, and reconnect with the deepest longings, intentions, and purposes of your life. Without question, it is one of the most important and transformative steps anyone can take on the journey through cancer.

Why is this so? The answer begins with an obvious but rarely acknowledged truth. Each of us hopes to get what we want in life and to avoid what we don't want. We all want pleasure, and we all want to avoid pain. We all want happiness and want to minimize suffering. Underlying the desire for happiness and pleasure is a fundamental desire for the experience of love and joy that is, ultimately, our true nature. We can say, therefore, that the foundation of all human behavior is, ultimately, the desire to know one's self.

In our everyday lives these ideas are rarely acknowledged. We are all so busy, who has the time? Without really thinking about it, we continue to plunge ahead each day, doing the things we hope and believe will bring us pleasure and make us happy—or help us to avoid suffering and pain.

What makes human beings so unique, and human endeavors so diverse, however, is that each of us has a different idea about what brings us happiness or what brings us pain. That's why some people exercise, or drink alcohol, or pursue a career, or go hiking in the mountains, or go dancing in nightclubs—and others don't. It's why some people become businessmen, some teachers, some parents, and others monks or priests. Nonetheless, underlying all of these activities is the same impulse to seek happiness and pleasure, to avoid pain and suffering, and ultimately to experience love and joy. It is the same impulse that compels people to seek medical help when they are diagnosed with a serious illness.

Virtually every cancer patient I have seen is, at least initially, experiencing some kind of physical, mental, emotional, or spiritual pain. In many patients, the distress is most acute at the moment of their diagnosis. As we have discussed, few words in our culture create a bigger avalanche of pain, confusion, and fear than the words "I'm sorry, but you have cancer."

Remarkably, the mental, emotional, and spiritual pain that most cancer patients experience far exceeds their physical pain. This has become even more true in recent years, as advances in screening and diagnosis have led increasingly to the detection of cancer long before the onset of any physical symptoms.

Some cancers present with an unremittant cough, blood in the urine, or an ache in the upper abdomen. Many more are detected by an abnormal blood test, an abnormal mammogram, a small and completely painless lump, or a swollen lymph node. Quite often, patients believed they were in perfect health. *They had no idea they had cancer.*

Regardless of the type of cancer or the stage at the time of diagnosis, the degree of mental, emotional and spiritual pain is often the same. In a huge number of cases, it is actually the pain and fear *associated* with cancer, rather than any specific physical symptoms, that causes people to seek medical help.

Certainly patients come to physicians because they want to "get rid of their cancer" as quickly and as easily as possible. But on a deeper level, they also want help in changing how they *feel*. Often they are confused. Often they feel overwhelmed. Almost always, they are deeply afraid.

Doctors must understand that patients want them not only to get rid of their disease and take away their physical pain, but to *take away their fear as well*. When physicians realize that their role is not only to address clinical symptoms, but also to help patients and family members feel better at *every level* of their being, an important step will be taken toward fulfilling the ultimate, as well as the relative, purpose of medicine.

What is the best way to fulfill both of these purposes? In this book we have explored a number of the key elements, and in this chapter we will explore another important one. Level Six of this program, called *Life Assessment*, describes a process for identifying the meaning and purpose of your life, clarifying specific goals for the coming year, and considering how you wish to be remembered after you are gone. These are essential, invaluable distinctions for patients and family members.

LIFE ASSESSMENT

Amid all of the effort and activity that takes place in helping cancer patients to prolong their lives, two questions are almost never asked of them. The first is: "Do you really want to live?" and the second is: "If so, *why?*"

Most people respond to these questions as if the answer were self-evident: *Of course I want to live.* This is a basic, human, and understandable response. Throughout nature, after all, life resists death. But when asked exactly *why* they want to live, many patients don't know how to respond. This is usually because no one has ever asked them this question before, or they have never asked it of themselves. Some break down in tears as they realize they don't really know the answer. Others are puzzled and become curious. A few become hostile, outraged to be asked such a thing.

The Dalai Lama of Tibet has explored these questions in terms of humanity as a whole and has stated with clarity and elegance: "All beings want to be happy." But finding happiness is often not as simple as it appears.

We all know that people seek happiness in many different ways, yet the desired result frequently remains elusive. We look to our careers, our children, our relationships, or in a thousand other places for fulfillment and happiness. Sometimes it appears to work, at least for a while. At other times the activities we pursue only lead us to more pain. Despite this almost universal experience, few people take the time to assess whether the way they are living their lives *will ever* really bring them the happiness they seek. Tragically, in their efforts to find happiness in external things and conditions, they lose sight of their deeper needs and priorities and their true meaning and purpose.

When people are diagnosed with cancer these deeper issues can instantly and dramatically rise to the surface. Basic changes invariably begin to occur in how patients perceive their lives. Everything that had been taken for granted is now no longer certain—including how much longer they may expect to live. In this context, many things that were previously regarded as significant or even essential may, in one moment, not look that way anymore at all.

Prior to getting cancer, most of our hopes and fears in life are focused in the external world. A cancer diagnosis immediately shifts attention inward. An important reason for this is that cancer instantly and forever shatters the illusion of immortality. The collective, unspoken dream that we have "all the time in the world" is now gone. In its place often comes an entirely new set of questions: *What do I really care about? What is the real meaning and purpose of my life? What are my most important goals?* And also, *How do I want to be remembered after I am gone from this life?*

As this process of inquiry begins, patients have an opportunity to discover—or rediscover—what is most important to them. It is a chance to identify their true purpose in life and begin moving immediately in the direction of fulfilling it.

There are three very important reasons why finding clear and coherent answers to these questions is so important on the journey through cancer:

FIRST: CANCER OFTEN BRINGS ABOUT DIFFICULT AND CHALLENGING TIMES. This is especially true of advanced or aggressive cancers, particularly those that cannot be easily cured with surgery. When you know exactly why you want to live, you have a clear and personally compelling motivation for fighting on. You are able to focus on *reasons for living*, rather than on whatever might not be going well at the moment.

Friedrich Nietzsche wrote, "He who has an important enough *why* can bear almost any *how*." We have all heard stories of patients who were given only a few weeks to live but defied their doctors' predictions and survived to be present at a wedding, graduation, or anniversary celebration months later. Some patients live years longer than expected. While many factors influence the outcome of stories like these, it is clear that the patients benefited from well-defined and compelling reasons for living.

SECOND: ON THE JOURNEY THROUGH CANCER YOU WILL HAVE DIMINISHED RESOURCES OF TIME AND ENERGY. As we have seen, cancer challenges patients and family members on many levels. Dealing with the logistical elements of cancer care consumes valuable resources of time, money, emotional energy, and physical strength. This may persist through treatment, and sometimes even beyond. As a result, cancer patients simply cannot afford unfulfilling or destructive thoughts, activities, and relationships. Many people find that cancer is the catalyst for long-avoided changes. Some people finally stop smoking or drinking, change their diet, and start exercising. For others, it might mean reconsidering or completely changing a job or career. It might also mean changing or even ending a relationship, or beginning a new one. And for some patients, the experience of cancer will cause them to begin to examine and explore some of their deepest beliefs and ideas about why they are alive.

THIRD: SOME PEOPLE WILL DISCOVER THAT THEY DON'T REALLY WANT TO FIGHT THEIR DISEASE. Patients may feel, for whatever reason, that they are unwilling to undergo surgery, radiation, or chemotherapy, or even alternative or complementary approaches to healing. After reflecting on their situation, some people feel that they have lived a good life and are ready to let go. Others may come to the same conclusion but by a very different route. They may feel that life has been a difficult or even an exhausting experience. They have suffered, and struggled, perhaps for a long time, and they don't wish to make any further efforts to keep living.

Unfortunately, in our society this perspective is rarely supported. All too often, patients endure arduous medical procedures and treatments because they are simply not clear about what they truly want to do. Rarely are they helped to explore these issues in the most open, supportive, and conscious way.

There are other instances in which patients are indeed clear about what they want to do, but they can't *give themselves permission* to let go. They're forbidden to do so by their religious beliefs or their cultural training. Or the medical environment in which they find themselves may not support such a decision. Except for the most elderly, the most frail, and the most infirm, our culture gives very, very few people permission to say, "I want to die." Great shame is attached to feeling this way, let alone saying it outright. From both a moral as well as a medical-legal perspective, it is usually considered to be hugely insensitive, if not outright criminal, even to suggest that it might be in someone's best interest to end their struggle to keep the physical body alive. I want to clarify that, in pointing this out, I am not advocating physician-assisted suicide or euthanasia. In my experience as a physician, and especially as an oncologist, I have seen very few patients who could not be made comfortable with appropriate care and adequate doses of medications. I am speaking here only of supporting a patient's right to decline treatment for any disease, even if the refusal seems unreasonable to us, and even if it hastens his or her death.

Perhaps most tragic of all are people with advanced cancer who are truly prepared to die, have given themselves permission and are at peace with their choice, *and* have the support of their physician—but can't let go because of pressure from family members. The family is unable and unwilling to face their own unresolved pain, grief, guilt, or anger, so the patient must suffer through tears, pleas, and guilt.

Gloria Parker was a sixty-eight-year-old woman with an advanced ovarian cancer that kept progressing after a number of different treatments. When she came to my office for a scheduled follow-up visit, she was exhausted. In fact, she was dying, but her family would not accept it. Over the weekend her four children had flown in from different parts of the country. They all had ideas of what was wrong with her, what was wrong with her medical care, and what should be done to "turn this situation around." One of her daughters, a strict vegetarian, wanted her to immediately start a macrobiotic diet. A second daughter was convinced that her mother was "starving to death," and demanded to know why I wouldn't give her high-dose intravenous vitamins, which she was sure would save her life. One of her sons wanted to fly her immediately to the Memorial Sloan-Kettering Cancer Center in New York City, certain that "they will have something to offer that you don't." Another son wanted to take her to a clinic in Tijuana, Mexico, that he heard had "great success" in curing cancer with herbs and coffee enemas. Meanwhile, Mrs. Parker's husband was out in the parking lot, crying.

Mrs. Parker herself was getting weaker and weaker, and was starting to feel short of breath. She was gravely ill, and a decision had to be made about what to do. As we started to discuss the options, she told me that she understood what was happening and that she did not want to do anything more to prolong her life. She told me very clearly and serenely that she was "ready to go." I asked her if she wanted to go home to die, or if she would prefer to go into the hospital. She said, "Please, put me in the hospital, because my family is driving me crazy. They won't let me die in peace. I'm ready to go, but they won't let me."

THE LIFE-ASSESSMENT PROCESS

We have covered many important issues in the preceding pages. To help patients address these issues, I ask them to begin by responding in writing to some basic questions:

- What is the meaning and purpose of your life?
- What are your most important goals for the next year?
- How do you want to be remembered after you are gone?

In the balance of this chapter, we'll look at these questions one by one.

1. What is the meaning and purpose of your life?

As we have discussed, a diagnosis of cancer often irrevocably shatters the illusion of immortality that so many of us harbor. For many cancer patients and their loved ones, this marks one of the most important turning points in their lives. As the illusion of immortality shatters, an opening can occur—a unique opportunity in which to explore some of the deepest and most important questions of life.

In the life-assessment process, patients' responses to the question *What is the meaning and purpose of your life?* are often referred to as *mission* statements. They actually include three distinct but closely related components: the *purpose* of your life, your *mission* in life, and the *vision* you may hold for your life. These three concepts—*purpose, mission,* and *vision*—are often confused in people's minds. But the distinctions between them can be critical, particularly for someone on the journey through cancer.

If I may use myself as an example, I would say, most succinctly, that the *purpose* of my life is *to know and celebrate my true Self—the timeless, eternal essence of God, of spirit, and of all beings—and to be a powerful presence of love, joy, wisdom, compassion, awareness, and truth for myself and others.* These are the values that inspire me most deeply and call to my heart, again and again and again. These are the qualities that I aspire to understand and embody in my life. And these are the ideals that bring me the greatest experience of love, joy, and fulfillment in life.

It has been humorously said, "At the end of your life, God will not ask you, '*Why didn't you spend more time at the office?*'"—and there is real wisdom in this. I am convinced that at the end of *my* life the questions that will matter most to me are: *Did I come to know my true Self? Did I live and embody the highest truths and values I discovered? Did I share the gifts that were given to me? Did I live my life as fully as possible? And, above all, did I love—myself as well as others—as fully and completely as possible?*

You may notice that my purpose in life includes no mention of my work as a physician or my specialty as an oncologist. My *mission,* however, is to create a new paradigm of medicine that promotes awareness, healing, and transformation at the deepest levels of the body, mind, heart, and spirit of all beings. It is clear to me that the ultimate purpose of this new paradigm of medicine is *to assist all beings to experience unbounded love and joy, and to know that this is the essence of who we all truly are.* This is the gift I want to bring forth and share with the world. This is the mission I want to accomplish while I am alive on this earth.

Finally, my *vision* is the worldly expression of my mission. My own personal vision is to see this new paradigm of medicine made available to everyone in the world. My vision, therefore, is the tangible and full realization of my mission.

Cancer patients and their family members—like many other people—are often not clear about the important distinctions between their *purpose, mission,* and *vision.* Achieving clarity about these issues can be life-transforming, and this was certainly true for Beverly Martin, the woman with breast cancer we met in chapter 2.

When Beverly underwent a modified radical mastectomy and axillary lymph node dissection, the tumor was found to have spread to thirteen of her nineteen axillary lymph nodes. Following her surgery, Beverly was advised by several leading medical centers to undergo conventional dose adjuvant chemotherapy, followed thereafter by high-dose chemotherapy and stem-cell rescue. This would not have been easy for anyone to accept, but it was even harder for Beverly, an otherwise healthy and vibrant woman who had "barely taken an aspirin" in her entire life. She'd had no prior illnesses or surgeries, and before the discovery of her breast cancer all of her encounters with the health care system were completely routine and unremarkable.

Her experiences following her breast cancer diagnosis had been quite traumatic for her. It was at this stage of her journey through cancer that Beverly and I had our first talk on the phone. Our conversation that day prompted her initial visit to see me at my cancer center in Florida.

I have a vivid memory of her first visit. Beverly had a quiet but striking intensity. Within a few minutes of meeting her, it was absolutely clear that she wanted to do everything possible to overcome her fears and conquer her disease. As I began to talk with her and her husband, Jeff, it also became clear that she brought this same intensity to all areas of her life.

Underlying her determination was the honest, very human fear that I'd heard in our first telephone conversation. Beverly's husband was also struggling with that fear. They were both successful people and were used to being in control of their lives. In fact, in most situations they were used to helping others. Now *they* were the ones who needed help, and everything seemed to be coming unhinged.

Our initial visit covered a wide range of topics, including the serious nature of her breast cancer. Beverly understood the risks of her situation and she was determined to do everything she could to help hearself. Although she certainly did not wish to abandon conventional medicine, she was also interested in pursuing any alternative and complementary modalities that might be of benefit to her. We discussed a variety of options, and she asked me what I would do in her situation. I answered her question honestly and gave her some extra advice to think about before she made any final decisions, as she and her husband went off for a brief vacation.

About a week later, Beverly called and told me that she and Jeff had decided to take my advice and go through conventional chemotherapy, followed by radiation. She had also decided that she would consider having further treatment with high-dose chemotherapy and stem-cell transplant, but not until the first part of her treatment was done.

Beverly also said that she wanted to do *everything else* she could to help herself heal at all levels. Would it be possible for her and Jeff to move to Vero Beach so she could have her treatment at my center? She wanted to go through the entire seven-level program, and Jeff was very supportive of the idea. What did I think?

I told her I thought it was a terrific idea, and that I would be honored to have her as a patient.

Several days later, Beverly and Jeff arrived and were ready to get started. We reviewed all of the medical aspects of her case and discussed the details of her proposed chemotherapy treatments. The numerous logistical questions about all the aspects of her medical care were addressed and answered, and arrangements were made for her to receive her first chemotherapy treatment in two days.

After going through all of the technical issues, I asked Beverly and Jeff if they *both* wanted to participate in the entire seven-level program. Beverly was enthusiastic, but Jeff was less so, although he did offer his full support to Beverly's participation. He also agreed to take part to the extent that he felt comfortable and interested.

I have found it is best if patients and their spouses engage in this entire program together, with equal interest and focus. However, this is not always possible, nor is it absolutely required. Even if the patient alone participates, everyone benefits.

Toward the end of our first visit, I asked Beverly if she was ready to start the program. She said, "You bet!"

I then asked if she would be willing to take a few minutes to write out an answer to one of the questions in our "homework packet." This is part of the materials used by patients and family members as they go through the program. She again quickly agreed, and I took a sheet of paper from the packet and handed it to her. At the top of the page were spaces for her name, the date, and another space to indicate which "version" of the document this would be, since her responses might change over time. Below was a single statement: *"The meaning and purpose of my life is…"* followed by a number of blank lines in which to write her answer.

I watched as Beverly silently read, with Jeff looking over her shoulder. "Dr. Geffen," she said after a few moments, "I have no idea how to answer this. It would take me all day! I have never really thought about this before."

"That's completely understandable and okay," I replied. "Don't feel like you have to write a Ph.D. thesis, or that you've got to express yourself perfectly. We'll be revisiting this question periodically during the program, and your answer may change with time. But for now, all that matters is that we get started and see what comes up. Are you willing to do that?"

"All right," Beverly said, closing her eyes.

"Take a few deep breaths," I said, "and begin to look inside yourself, maybe deeper now than ever before. Exhale slowly, and relax. Begin to go into your heart, and ask yourself, 'What am I here to do?' 'What do I really want to accomplish while I am alive?' *What is the real meaning and purpose of my life?*"

I watched Beverly's face as she began to ask herself these questions. I've had the privilege of facilitating this process with patients and family members many times, but seeing it happen is always captivating. People are often frustrated at first, as Beverly was. They're concerned about finding the "right" answer, when there's really no such thing as a "wrong" one.

After a few moments, I asked Beverly if she was ready to write an answer to the question. She opened her eyes and firmly nodded her head, and I saw that she was indeed ready. "The most important thing," I reminded her, "is to write freely and spontaneously, without editing too much or trying to make it absolutely perfect. Later we can go back and see if it makes sense to you."

Beverly picked up the pen and began writing. A few minutes later she handed me the page, on which were written the following three sentences:

My mission is to validate battered women by providing support and information to them in court and in crisis intervention teams established within our country. This mission is not limited to New Jersey, and it has no time constraints. As long as there is inequality between people, my mission is incomplete.

Beverly watched anxiously as I read her mission statement. "Thank you for sharing this with me, Beverly," I said. "Would you be willing to read it out loud, so Jeff can hear it, too?"

After a moment of hesitation, Beverly said, "Sure."

For many people, reading their mission statement is an act of unaccustomed and perhaps uncomfortable self-revelation. It is also—very often—a moment of great revelation for the spouse.

After Beverly finished reading her statement, I thanked her again for sharing it. Then I said, "This mission statement tells me so much about you. Would you like me to tell you what I learned?"

"Oh, yes," she replied. I then described for her the person I saw reflected in her mission statement. In just the first two sentences it was clear that Beverly was a person who was deeply concerned and moved by the problems experienced by abused women. She was a person who was motivated to *action*. She was someone who not only cared about the plight of others, but who also wanted to *do* something about it. Furthermore, she was willing to "think big." Her mission was not limited to her home state, and was subject to "no time constraints." As with the treatment of her breast cancer, she was willing to do whatever it took to accomplish her goals.

I was somewhat disturbed, however, by the third sentence of her mission statement: *"As long as there is inequality between people, my mission is incomplete."*

There was no question that Beverly was committed to alleviating injustice and inequality in the world, and she was also willing to commit herself over the long term to helping resolve these issues on earth. Unfortunately her commitment was expressed in a way that seemed to eliminate any chance that it would ever be fulfilled. Although I consider myself a naturally optimistic person, it seems to me that there very likely will be *some* "inequality between people" on earth for a very long time to come. Based on what Beverly had written, there was no way she could ever achieve the sense of accomplishment and fulfillment that she so clearly desired, and deserved.

"Beverly," I said, "would you like some feedback from me about your mission statement?"

"Yes, absolutely," she replied. "Please tell me what you think."

I related some of the positive impressions I had gained from reading her statement. "Yet," I continued, "I am a bit concerned about your last sentence. Now, I do believe that the world is evolving and getting better. However, it seems to me that there might be *some* inequality between people for a really long time. If so, isn't it possible that you could work your entire life and never fulfill your mission?"

"Yes," she said quietly, "but it doesn't matter, because I have to fight this battle no matter what. I have to keep trying."

"Beverly, I know that's true for you, and I completely understand. In fact, your determination about this is very inspiring, and I want to help you find the strength to accomplish all of your goals. But I'm just as committed to helping you find inner fulfillment as a human being—regardless of whether this external struggle is lost or won."

"What do you mean?" she asked.

"Well, what we do in life is extremely important to most of us and can be very fulfilling and rewarding. However, sometimes we make an effort for many years and our 'worldly goals' are not achieved. Or sometimes they are achieved, and we still don't find the happiness and fulfillment we seek. I believe it is very important—particularly when you are dealing with a situation like cancer—that you commit yourself to finding and experiencing the deepest levels of love, joy, and fulfillment you really want, each and every day, *independent* of the things you want to do in the world. To a great extent, none of us can really control what happens outside of ourselves, so we've got to find the happiness we seek *inside* of ourselves—even as we continue to fight the battles that we have chosen to fight, and to work on changing the things that we believe are important to change. This is true with cancer, too. It is *especially* true with cancer. You can do everything right, even perfectly, and it may not turn out the way you want. So along the way, each and every day, it's important that you find and experience the love and joy you truly want."

"How do I do that, Dr. Geffen?" Beverly asked. "What else should I do now?"

"For now, Beverly, what you have done is absolutely beautiful, and certainly enough for today. You've taken a huge step forward, and I want to give you time to let this process unfold naturally. On your next visit, we'll talk some more. In the meantime, when you think about our meeting today, ask yourself how you might begin to experience a deeper sense of fulfillment, here and now, as you and Jeff go through this journey together."

Beverly and Jeff thanked me, and they left with a stack of information about her treatment. They also had a plan of action for exploring the deeper dimensions of healing her body, mind, heart, and spirit. This included getting a better understanding of her upcoming chemotherapy treatments and joining one of our support groups. It also included a plan to begin thinking of and nourishing her body as if it were a garden rather than a machine. She would be evaluating her food and exercise, joining a yoga class, and getting a massage at least once or twice a week, particularly just before her chemotherapy treatments. Jeff agreed to schedule a massage for himself and to accompany Beverly to the support group. They agreed to spend some time together each day, alone—with no TV, radio, newspaper, or any other distractions—just simply being together and sharing what was going on for each of them. I asked Beverly to purchase a bound journal and spend at least ten or fifteen minutes each day, quietly, writing down whatever thoughts, feelings, and questions might come to her. She would also be signing up for a meditation class the next day.

Over the next week, Beverly and Jeff were in the cancer center every day, participating in various components of the seven-level program. She received her first cycle of chemotherapy without any problems and had many conversations with our staff, other patients and their family members, and with our support group leader. During these discussions, the question occasionally arose, "Why do you want to help other women? Why do you want to do so much for others?"

Her answers always led to the same place. "Because it makes me happy to do things for other people," she said. "It brings me joy. It also helps me to grow and to understand myself better."

Beverly and I had a formal follow-up visit a week after our first meeting. After reviewing her medical status and her progress with the seven levels of the program, we turned again to her personal mission statement.

"Well, Beverly," I said, "are you ready to go to the next level with your mission statement?"

"Sure," she replied. "What do I have to do?"

"It's simple. We're just going to go through the same process as before. Only now you've gotten over some of your fears about cancer and about chemotherapy. You also have some more experience in getting quiet and going inside of yourself. As a result, you might be able to hear what your heart is trying to say to you now in a different way than before. Are you ready?"

"Yes."

"Okay," I began. "Once again, close your eyes and take a few deep breaths. Let yourself begin to relax, and go inside. Go deep into your heart, deep into yourself, and ask, *'What is the real meaning and purpose of my life?'*"

As she closed her eyes and looked silently into her heart, I reminded Beverly that the key was to allow whatever thoughts, feelings, and ideas that were inside of her to emerge without any stress or strain. She needed only to listen intently to her own inner voice and express freely and spontaneously whatever she heard. There was no need to get it "perfect."

A few minutes later she composed the following second draft of her mission statement:

> *It is my mission to heal and benefit from this healing experience spiritually; to learn and grow emotionally; and to mature with a new understanding of myself. It is with this new enlightened self that I will gain joy and peace in my heart by giving to others, in service to those who need support.*

In just one week, the change from the first mission statement was unmistakable and dramatic. Beverly was now committed to growing and healing, emotionally and spiritually, regardless of her circumstances. She was also getting closer to actually seeing the distinction between her true *purpose* in life and her *mission* and *vision* of helping women who were suffering from abuse. She now had a mission statement that gave her, both consciously and unconsciously, a much greater chance of experiencing love, joy, and fulfillment on an *ongoing basis*, with much less dependence on outside circumstances. The language of her mission statement still revealed her longing to serve, support, and care for other human beings. This was not surprising since it was such a strong part of Beverly's character.

When I asked her about the changes in what she'd written, Beverly was bubbling over with excitement. She no longer felt she had to "save the world" in order to be happy and fulfilled. She didn't feel any less concern for the plight of abused women, but somehow a huge burden had been lifted from her shoulders. She was no longer willing to let events in the external world determine whether she was happy and fulfilled.

A week later, on her third follow-up visit, we went through the mission statement process again. After closing her eyes and going deeply into her heart, Beverly wrote her third, and final, draft.

> *The purpose of my life is to experience abundant love, joy, and peace in my heart, and to experience physical, mental, emotional, and spiritual health and freedom, and to share this with others.*

Reading this, I sensed Beverly had now really connected to her *true* purpose, which was to experience "abundant love, joy, and peace in my heart," rather than "trying to save the world." She also wanted to experience "physical, mental, emotional, and spiritual health and freedom," and she knew she could move in this direction every day of her life. She was no longer asking for "perfection," and her fulfillment as a person no longer had anything to do with the conditions of the world. She realized that love, joy, and freedom can exist even in the presence of imperfection and challenge. And in the midst of all of this, the same deep and compelling impulses to share and give to others were once again expressed.

"How do you feel about this mission statement?" I asked Beverly.

She looked at me with her eyes wide, glowing, and excited. "I feel great about it, Dr. Geffen," she said. "It's so simple and so clear. And I can live this and experience it every single day. It all lies within myself, within *me*. There is such a tremendous feeling of strength and freedom in realizing this. Thank you for helping me to see this, and to understand."

2. What are your most important goals for the next year?

The next phase of the process of self-discovery in Level Six has to do with clearly defining—and prioritizing—your most important goals. Few people ever take the time to write down their specific goals, or to establish meaningful time frames for achieving them—just as they rarely take the time to identify and understand their true life purpose. These issues can become very important on the journey through cancer, for a variety of reasons. In order to illustrate this, let's look at the following example.

Kate Seymour is a sixty-two-year-old woman from Michigan who was diagnosed with low-grade non-Hodgkin's lymphoma three years ago. At the time of her diagnosis she had fairly extensive Stage IV disease and underwent aggressive treatment with chemotherapy. The treatment was quite difficult for her, but she got through it and achieved a complete remission of her disease, which lasted for two years. About a year ago her lymphoma recurred, and she subsequently underwent evaluation and treatment at several different medical centers around the country. Each time she was treated her enlarged lymph nodes would shrink, but then they would start to grow again. This scenario is quite common for low-grade non-Hodgkin's lymphomas. Many patients can be successfully treated on and off like this for a number of years, especially now that a variety of new treatments for non-Hodgkin's lymphoma have become available.

Kate's husband, Ron, was totally devoted to her. Like Kate, he was also very devoted to their twenty-eight-year-old daughter, who had Down's syndrome and lived in a residential home in New York State. From the time of Kate's initial cancer diagnosis Ron had accompanied her on all her medical evaluations and treatments, and did everything he could to help care for her and manage the affairs of their family.

The past year had been especially difficult for both of them: for Kate because of all the treatments she had undergone, and for Ron because of all the work he had to do to get everything organized and stay on track. They were both extremely tired from the ordeal they had been through.

Kate and Ron came to see me because she strongly believed that there must be "more that I can do to help myself other than just keep taking chemotherapy." Like Beverly, and like so many people with cancer, she didn't want to abandon conventional medicine. She just wanted to *do more*. The problem was that she didn't know *what more to do*, and she didn't know where to find clear, coherent, and reliable advice.

At our first meeting we went through an extensive standard medical evaluation for Kate. Over the previous month a number of lymph nodes in her abdomen had started to enlarge, and these were now causing her to experience abdominal pain and swelling. It was evident she needed additional treatment, and she was ready and willing to follow my recommendations.

But again, she wanted *more* than just chemotherapy. She wanted to explore the entire seven-level program that she had heard about from friends.

After Kate's medical plan was established, I asked her and Ron, as I had done with Beverly and her husband, if they *both* wanted to participate in the program. I was happy when Ron agreed.

I then guided them both through the mission statement process. After they were done writing, I asked them if they would read their mission statements to each other, and they agreed.

Here is Kate's mission statement:

> *The meaning and purpose of my life is to have a loving, close-knit family that is cemented together with a strong faith in God, in whose footsteps I hope to follow. First and foremost is my strong relationship with Ron, and then my children and grandchildren, which give meaning and purpose to my life.*

Ron's eyes filled with tears as he heard Kate read her mission statement. I have to say that this is an almost universal phenomenon. When people share their deepest thoughts and feelings about what is most important to them in life in this way—especially to those whom they love very much—an outpouring of love occurs *almost every single time* that is something extraordinary to behold. Facilitating this process for individuals and families is one of the things I most love about my work.

Here is Ron's mission statement:

> *The meaning and purpose of my life is to be a steadfast and consistent support and provider for my wife and family; to make a productive and positive contribution to the society and environment in which I live; to be a devoted and dependable follower of God's word; to try to live each day to the fullest and minimize regrets; to*

be self-reliant but not proud; to recognize and accept help when offered and needed; and to appreciate all that has been given me.

As one might have expected, when Kate heard Ron read his mission statement, she couldn't help but cry.

Kate and Ron were inspired by the mission statement process and wanted to keep going. So I handed them the next page in the homework packet. At the top was a space for name, date, and which version of their answers the page would contain. Below this information was the statement: *My top twenty goals for the next year are…*

When they read this, they exclaimed, "Oh my goodness! What a concept!"

"Kate and Ron," I said, "I'm going to ask you to think about your top twenty goals for the next year, and in a few minutes I'll ask you to write them down. But first, there are a few ground rules that are important to understand that will help you get the most out of this process.

"First of all, when I ask you to begin writing down your goals, I want you to write down whatever comes into your mind, *without editing it.* This is really very important. Your mind may have a tendency to say things like, 'Oh, this is unreasonable,' or 'I can't do that,' or 'This is *impossible.*' If you notice that happening, try to ignore it, and write down whatever you were thinking anyway. The main thing at this point is to not edit or filter your goals in any way. Just write down whatever comes to your mind, no matter how crazy or ridiculous you may think it is. We can talk about your goals later, but for now, I just want you to get them out and written down on paper.

"The next thing is, I want you to *keep on writing* whatever comes to your mind until you get to the end of the page. If your mind goes blank, and you don't know what to write, allow yourself to think of some things that you would really love to do or experience. Ask yourself, '*What would make me feel really good to do or experience in the next year?*' And then, just write it down—once again, whether or not you think it is reasonable, crazy, or even possible. Okay?"

They both nodded their agreement, but then Kate asked me a question.

"Why do you want to know these things?"

"That's a great question," I replied, "and I'll answer it for you precisely.

But first, let me ask you both something. You have come to me for help, correct?"

"Yes," they both agreed.

"And you want my input about how to best help Kate fight this lymphoma, feel better, and live as long as possible, right?"

"Yes, exactly," they both said, almost in unison.

"Well, in order to give you the best possible advice, *I need to know what your goals are.* To begin with, I'd like to know what your goals are for the next year. I want to know what you are fighting for, what you want to accomplish, and what you want to experience—*specifically*—in the next year. It's important to know these things because it might influence so many things, like what kind of treatment we use for your lymphoma, or when we do it, or how we might want or need to schedule some breaks in your treatment. If I don't know what your goals are, then how can I help you fulfill them?"

"Wow," Ron replied. "That is amazing. No one ever asked us anything like this before."

"But, Dr. Geffen," Kate asked, "are you suggesting that I will only live for another year?"

"Absolutely not," I replied. "I'm not suggesting that at all. I can't tell you how long you are going to live. In fact, no one can, really. We've just met each other, and I still don't know how well you are going to respond to your next treatments. You might live a very long time, or less than a very long time. No one can really know for sure right now. But I want to have an idea of what your priorities are for the next year, so we have a place to start, and plan, and have some real goals to work toward and look forward to.

"Now, I'm not saying that you will necessarily meet or fulfill *every single one* of your goals in the next year, but at least we can take a look and see what they are. If you *are* meeting some of your goals along the way—and especially if they are some of *the most important ones*—you are much more likely to feel better than if none of your most important goals are being met. Wouldn't you say that is true?"

After thinking about my question, they nodded in agreement.

"Also," I went on, "having a list of your specific goals, which we will be reviewing periodically throughout your treatment, will help keep you focused on what is *most important* for you to be doing. It will help keep you from getting sidetracked or distracted by things that are bound to come up along the way, but that aren't really *that* important. Does this make sense?"

"Yes," they replied.

"Great. Because there is actually another great thing this list can give you."

"What's that?" they asked.

"Well, if you encounter any really rough times along the way, this list can be helpful in reminding you *why* you have chosen to keep fighting your disease. Sometimes, if things get tough, you can forget why you're doing this. It is very human, and natural, and common. But if that happens, each of you will be able to pull out your list and remember exactly what you are fighting for. Does that make sense to you?"

"Yes," they said. "Let's get started."

I then asked them to close their eyes for a few minutes and settle into their hearts. I asked them to take a few deep breaths and to start visualizing all the things they wanted to do in the coming year. I reminded them not to edit anything, just to see and feel all the things that inspired them, things that they would like to do and experience, no matter how mundane or even obvious those things might be. Then I asked them to open their eyes and start writing.

After several minutes of writing Kate and Ron looked up from their pages and indicated to me that they were done. I then asked each of them to read their list out loud.

Here is Kate's list of goals:

My top 20 goals for the next year are...
1. To become healthy, strong, and energetic
2. Not to worry or be fearful—and to have a positive attitude
3. To take one day at a time
4. To find joy in every day
5. Have a family reunion in Colorado at a nice ranch
6. Take a trip to Antigua with Ron
7. Visit my children and grandchildren
8. Take time each day to read the Bible
9. Go on a fishing trip
10. Have a calmer relationship with my mother

11. Stop looking like a cancer patient
12. Find tranquillity of spirit
13. Be more involved with Carol [her daughter] and Pathfinder Village [a residential home for children with Down's syndrome]
14. Play golf again
15. Be more at peace with life
16. Take more trips exploring the Northeast
17. Plan a reunion with Sally [her best friend from childhood]
18. Feel strong enough to hike
19. Take an interest in cooking and having friends for dinner
20. Have more courage in the face of adversity

After Kate finished reading her list, I asked Ron how he felt hearing Kate's goals for the year.

"It's a big list," he said. "It's very ambitious. I didn't know she wanted to do all those things."

"But how does it make you *feel* to hear all those things she wants to do?" I asked again.

"Well, it makes me feel excited, and happy. It's a lot to look forward to. But it also makes me a bit worried."

"Why?" I asked.

"Well, is she going to be strong enough to do all those things? Also, I don't know if *I* have the strength to do all those things, or to get them all organized."

These were important and legitimate things for Ron to wonder about, and I commended him for being so open and honest. I also wanted to address his concerns to put his mind at ease.

"John, we don't know if Kate will be strong enough to do everything on her list. We're going to look at the list in more detail a bit later, and she will decide what are the most important items for her to try and accomplish. So you don't necessarily have to worry about trying to get *everything* done.

"And you also don't have to feel responsible for fulfilling Kate's list. I know that you might naturally *feel* responsible, and I know that you will want to help her in any way that you can, but you are not actually responsible for that."

I then turned to Kate. "Is that true, Kate? Do you feel that Ron is responsible for fulfilling everything on your list in the next year?"

"Oh no," she replied, turning to her husband. "Ron, I love it that you always want to help me. But I don't want you to feel like you always have to do *everything*. I can help, too. And if I'm too tired, well, I'll just change the list, or we can get some other help. Okay?"

Ron looked visibly reassured.

"Great," I said. "Now, Ron, are you ready to read your list to Kate?"

He began reading. Here is Ron's list of goals:

My top 20 goals for the next year are...
 1. To support my wife and see her through this period of hardship
 2. Find time to learn how to paint better
 3. Become closer to my children and grandkids
 4. Find more time to fish
 5. Develop more patience
 6. Curtail feelings of anger
 7. Develop a keener understanding of life
 8. Better understand what is most important in life
 9. Maintain a sense of humor
10. Give more of myself to others
11. Play more golf
12. Handle frustrations, disappointments, and stress better
13. Be less selfish and introverted
14. Try to be a compassionate and good person
15. Maintain good health
16. Cheerfully step forward and give when asked
17. Try to do some volunteer work
18.
19.
20.

When Ron finished, I asked Kate how she felt hearing Ron's goals for the next year. She was very moved, and said so. She also said she was happy that some of his goals were to take care of himself and do things that he wanted to do. "Ron has sacrificed so much for me," she said. "I want him to do more for himself, too."

I noticed that Ron hadn't completed the last three goals on his list, and I asked him why.

"Well," he said. "I didn't want to fill them all in for myself. I wanted to leave room to find out what Kate's goals were, so I could help her fulfill some of them."

I was amazed at how completely devoted this man was to his wife. His love and concern for her was so apparent, and Kate was moved to tears when she heard Ron say why he had left his last three goals blank.

I asked Kate and Ron to look at their list and to renumber their goals with a red pen in order of priority. I then asked them both to rewrite their new lists on a clean goal sheet and read them out loud for each other once again.

One of the interesting things that came out of that process was a recognition by both Kate and Ron that the majority of their goals were very possibly attainable within the next year. Some of the goals were simple, others were more complex or challenging. But they realized that if they were committed, and if Kate's strength held up, there was a good chance they could accomplish most of them.

When I asked how they felt about having such a clear picture of what they wanted to accomplish, they both said they felt "great." They had a new sense of clarity and focus, and a renewed sense of determination of what they wanted to aim for. It was beautiful to see. They agreed to spend more time talking in the coming days to refine the priorities of their goals, and to find how they could work together to make sure that both of them felt that their goals were being pursued. For Ron, seeing Kate's goals written down gave him clarity on how he could really help her the most, which was so obviously his wish. Now he had an absolutely clear blueprint, written by her, of exactly what she wanted to accomplish in the next year, along with her commitment to communicating with him about how best to get there. For Kate, she now had a list of things that were important for Ron, written by him, which she could use to support him in taking care of himself as well.

Toward the end of our session, I had to ask Kate one last question. "I'm really curious about one thing," I said. "I noticed you said you wanted to take a trip to Antigua. Of all the places in the world, why do you want to go to Antigua?"

"Oh," Kate said, starting to blush. "Antigua is where Ron and I met, forty-one years ago. And that is where we went on our honeymoon. I have so many beautiful memories of being there. We haven't been there for so many years—and I thought, 'Wouldn't it be wonderful to go back again?'"

I looked at Ron, and he was smiling. No doubt he was recalling some of those same memories. "I haven't thought of that place for so long," he said. "But what a beautiful idea. If we can do it, let's go!"

Now I too was smiling. We talked about it some more, and agreed to make it a high priority for the coming year.

3. How do you want to be remembered?

A third part of the life-assessment process has to do with acknowledging the fact that at some time in the future we are all destined to die. This is true regardless of our circumstances in life. In the years I have spent working as an oncologist, I have found that it can be extremely powerful, inspiring, and revealing for cancer patients and their family members to take some time to think about how they want to be remembered after they are gone. Obviously this can be a sensitive subject for some people who are on the journey through cancer, because for them the reality of leaving may be closer than they might wish to acknowledge. Most cancer patients and their family members are also quite sensitive and attentive to any subtle nuances in their oncologists' words, tone of voice, facial expressions, and gestures. They often read much more into things that are said—or not said—in those interactions than is intended. As a result, I realize that asking a question such as *How do you want to be remembered?*" in an inappropriate or insensitive way—and without a clearly established context—might give the impression, or fear, that I think the patient might be dying soon.

However, when done properly and with sensitivity, helping patients and family members explore this question in a loving and supportive way can yield insights and breakthroughs that are moving, profound, and important.

This was true for Kate and Ron, who returned for a follow-up visit a week after our initial meeting. Kate had started a new chemotherapy regimen several days earlier. Her first treatment had gone well and over-all she felt quite stable. After I had carefully examined her, reviewed her lab results for the day, and addressed some additional questions about her treatment plan, they indicated to me that they were both eager to continue with the life-assessment process.

Kate and Ron shared with me that they had been spending time over the past week thinking about the meaning and purpose of their lives and talking more about their goals. This was bringing them closer in ways they had not anticipated, and they wanted to go further in understanding each other, and themselves.

We then reviewed their experience over the previous week and talked about some of the valuable insights they had gained from writing and sharing their personal mission statement and goals with each other.

"The next step of this process," I said, "is something I have also found to be very powerful and helpful for people. It raises a question that some of us may not want to look at, but it is a question that can lead to great insights into ourselves, and especially into the way we live our lives. Now, before we explore this, I want to ask you a different question. I'm curious about something, and maybe you can help me out.

"In the history of the world," I asked Kate and Ron, "since humans have been walking on the earth, how many people would you guess have lived, not counting the people who are alive right now?"

Kate and Ron gave me puzzled looks.

"Well," I said, "let's take a look. Right now, there are about six billion people alive on the earth. And we know that there are a *lot* more people alive today than ever before. True?"

"That seems right," they answered.

"Okay," I continued, "anthropologists estimate that since the beginning of human history there have been about ten billion people who have been alive on the earth, including everyone who is alive right now. Does that seem like a reasonable estimate?"

"I guess so," Kate and Ron said in unison.

"Okay. Now, of the ten billion people who ever lived, not counting the six billion who are alive today, how many does that leave?"

"About four billion people," Ron responded.

"That's right," I said. "And now, let me ask you another question. Of those four billion people who were alive before everyone who is alive now, what percentage of those people died?"

Kate and Ron then burst out laughing, and Kate said, "Well, *one hundred percent, of course!*"

"That's exactly right," I said. "And, if one hundred percent of the people who were ever alive in history before now died, what percentage of the people who are alive today do you think are likely to die at some point in the future?"

Again they laughed, and said, *"One hundred percent."*

"I would agree," I said. "Now, I guess it's possible that somebody, somewhere, has figured out how to never die, but I haven't run into that person yet! So, since one hundred percent of everyone who is alive today is likely to die at some point in the future, what do you think the likelihood is that—at some point in the future—*you and I* are also going to die?"

"Well, it's pretty certain," Kate said. "In fact, we're all going to die someday."

"Exactly," I said. "At least, it certainly looks that way right now. Anyway, I have another question. Since it seems likely that all of us are going to die at some point in the future, did you ever stop to think for a moment about how you'd like to be remembered after you are gone?"

They had never really stopped to think about it.

"Well," I continued, "most people don't really think about it. And sometimes, it's a shame. Because if they did, they might live their lives a bit differently."

"What do you mean?" they asked.

"I've talked to many people about this over the years," I said, "and I've always found it fascinating to explore with them how they want to be remembered after they're gone. I've also been very privileged, as you know, to have been able to serve as a guide for many people who are battling cancer, sometimes very aggressive cancer. It has been especially rewarding to explore these ideas with individuals who really recognize that they will not live forever. In these cases—quite often, but certainly not always—when people think about how they want to be remembered, they realize that they had better start doing some things differently, right now, or they may not be remembered in the way they truly want. And quite often, seeing this so clearly actually spurs them to make the changes they had really wanted to make in their lives all along.

"Another important benefit of this exploration," I went on, "is that it allows people an opportunity to think about the values and standards of behavior that they hold important in life. Knowing how you want to be remembered after you are gone can serve as sort of an inner-directed 'code of conduct,' which can help guide your decisions and actions *while you are alive*. This can be very helpful for anyone, especially anyone involved in the journey through cancer.

"Would you like to see how this works?" I asked.

"Yes," they replied. "We're ready."

I handed Kate and Ron a new piece of paper from the homework packet. Like the mission statement form, and the "Top 20 Goals for the Next Year" form, this page also had space at the top for their names, the date, and version number. Below that was the statement: *How and what I want to be remembered for in my life.*

Kate and Ron sat up straight in their chairs and prepared to begin the process.

"Okay," I said. "Let's begin by closing our eyes once again and taking a few deep breaths. I'd like you to begin to relax, as you've done before. I'd like you to start thinking about your life, and about the fact that—cancer or no cancer—someday you will be gone from this earth. When your time to go comes, and you have left, what are some of the things you would like people to say about you? How do you want to be remembered? What contributions do you want to have made? What kind of person do you want to have been? When your family, your children, your friends, and your colleagues think about you and speak about you after you're gone, what kind of person do you want them to say you were? Just go inside your heart right now, and listen to what your inner voice is saying. And when you feel ready, open your eyes, and start writing down whatever you feel about how and what you want to be remembered for in your life."

After a moment Kate and Ron each opened their eyes, and started writing. After several minutes they looked up at me again and indicated they were done.

"Great," I said. "Who would like to go first and read what they wrote?" Ron volunteered. Here is what he read, as Kate and I listened.

How and what I want to be remembered for in my life.
Ron Seymour was:
1. Someone who was trustworthy
2. A good husband
3. A good father
4. Somebody who could laugh at his own shortcomings
5. Someone who demonstrated compassion
6. Someone who was able to respect those who disagreed with him
7. Someone who could both work and play hard
8. A man who was true to his word
9. Someone who was a willing and generous giver of his time
10. A caring man

As Ron was reading, Kate's eyes filled with love and admiration.

"What do you think about what Ron wrote?" I asked.

"Well," she replied, "it is so moving for me to hear it, because what he wrote is *how he really is*. It's amazing. He really *is* all those things."

"How does it make you feel to hear that, Ron?" I asked.

"It feels very good," he replied. "I really try to be that kind of a person, but sometimes it's hard to know if I am succeeding." Then he became very quiet, almost withdrawn, and said, "I try very hard, but actually I often don't feel that I really am succeeding."

"Kate," I asked, "do you think Ron is succeeding?"

"Oh yes," she replied.

"Would you tell him directly?" I asked.

"Yes," she said, turning to Ron. "Ron, I want you to know how much I appreciate everything you do for me. And I want you to know how wonderful I think you are as a husband, as a father to our kids, and as a man."

Ron's eyes welled with tears. "Thank you," he said. "But you never told me that before."

This was followed by a long silence, as Kate thought about, and really heard, what he had said. Then, she said softly, "I'm so sorry, Ron. I didn't know you wanted me to tell you. You always seem so self-sufficient, and you never ask for anything. *So I thought you just knew.*"

"No," Ron replied, "I didn't know for sure. Sometimes I just want to be told. It feels good to hear you say it. Thank you."

A rich silence followed this interaction. After some time Kate said she felt ready to read her list. Here it is:

How and what I want to be remembered for in my life.
Kate Seymour was…
1. Someone who cared deeply for family
2. A loving wife
3. A caring mother and friend
4. A faithful servant of God
5. Someone who was nonjudgmental
6. Someone who had courage in the face of adversity
7. Someone who was sensitive to others' needs
8. A good listener
9. Someone who had a good sense of humor

After Kate finished reading, she and I both turned to Ron for his reaction. He was quiet, and I could tell he had been deeply moved. I asked Kate if she would read her list again, and she agreed.

Once again Ron remained quiet, as if it were hard for him to speak. He seemed a bit stunned. I looked at Kate's list and immediately noticed something that, intuitively, I felt was significant for Ron.

"Ron," I said gently, "are you aware that Kate said she wanted to be remembered first as someone who cared deeply for family, as a loving wife, and *then* as a caring mother and friend?"

"Yes," Ron replied quietly.

Something inside me felt inspired to look again at Kate's mission statement, which I had in hand. Immediately, my hunch was confirmed.

"Kate, would you be willing to read your mission statement out loud again?"

"You mean right now?" she asked.

"Yes," I replied.

"Sure," Kate said, and she again read aloud:

The meaning and purpose of my life is to have a loving, close-knit family that is cemented together with a strong faith in God, in

whose footsteps I hope to follow. First and foremost is my strong relationship with Ron, and then my children and grandchildren which give meaning and purpose to my life.

After she finished reading, I said, "Kate, would you read the second sentence one more time?"

"Okay," she replied, then read: *"First and foremost is my strong relationship with Ron, and then my children and grandchildren, which give meaning and purpose to my life."*

"Thank you, Kate," I said. "I have one more favor to ask. Would you be willing to read just the first part of that sentence one more time?"

"Sure," she said. *"First and foremost is my strong relationship with Ron."*

I looked at Ron, whose eyes were again filled with tears.

"Ron, how does it make you feel to hear what Kate has said? That she wants to be remembered as someone who cared deeply for family and as a loving wife, and *then* as a caring mother and friend?"

"It is amazing," Ron said.

"Why?" I asked.

"Because I never knew," he replied. "We've been married for forty-one years, *and I always thought I came second, after the kids.*"

"Kate," I said, "is that true? In your mind, and in your heart, does Ron come second?"

"Oh no," she said, turning to Ron. "I just thought you always knew, just like I thought you knew how much I appreciated you."

The look on both of their faces at that moment is impossible to describe. Love, sadness, joy, revelation, forgiveness, and gratitude were all mixed together. Something very deep, significant, and profound had occurred in the minds and hearts of these two courageous people. In their forty-one years together, it was—on some level—only in the past few minutes that they'd really seen and understood *how much* they loved each other, and how important they were to each other.

They hugged, and then looked into each other's eyes, which were filled with tears, tenderness, and love.

Very gently, I broke the silence. "Kate and Ron, I'd like to ask you one final question. What is it worth to you to know what you have discovered about each other and about your relationship today?"

They both looked at me and said, simultaneously, "It is worth every-thing...."

LETTING GO WHEN THE TIME IS RIGHT

As we discussed earlier in this chapter, the journey through cancer some-times brings people to very different conclusions about where they are in life, and how they might wish to proceed. Most truly wish to do all they can to keep living and to improve their situation. Some, however, come to a point in their journey where they realize that they do not have the will or desire to fight their disease—for whatever reason. When this occurs, I believe it is an important duty for us all to honor whatever choice an individual might make and to love them unconditionally.

When a person decides not to undertake a battle with his or her ill-ness, a different kind of opportunity arises, which can be sacred and pro-found. It is an opportunity to ask, "If I am going to die, what can I do right now to feel complete with my life? What do I need to do, or say, to those who have touched my life, so that I can die without any regrets or any fears? What do I need to do so that I can die with a full heart and a peaceful mind?"

Some people may need a great deal of assistance at such a critical time of their lives. Others might need help with only a few things. And still others may already feel complete, except for one issue that could touch any one of us. That issue is the simple fear of death itself.

The following story shows how this part of the journey through can-cer unfolded for one patient:

Mrs. Golashevsky was a lovely seventy-three-year-old Polish woman I was asked to see one day in the hospital for evaluation of newly diag-nosed colon cancer. Before entering her room I stopped to read her chart and learned some important things about her.

She lived alone in a small apartment and had not seen a doctor for many years. She and her husband had escaped from Poland after World

War Two to come to America. He had died two years earlier, and they had no children. After her husband's death she started visiting the local Polish American Club near her apartment, where she went regularly to eat. She had no other known relatives and only a few friends. One of those friends was a young Polish woman named Rachel Kosala who worked as a social worker and had brought Mrs. Golashevsky to the hospital two days before.

Several months ago, Mrs. Golashevsky started to feel tired and began to lose weight. She seemed more withdrawn than before and came to the club less often. A few friends noticed these changes and asked her if she was okay, but she would always say, "Yes, I'm fine. Thank you." A few weeks ago, she started to look quite pale. Again her friends asked if she was okay, and she said, "Thank you, really, I'm fine."

A week ago she stopped coming to the club altogether. This was highly unusual, and her friends became alarmed. They tried calling her at home, but got no answer. No one had ever been to her apartment before, and they didn't dare go uninvited. So they called Rachel and told her what was going on.

Rachel took the initiative to go to Mrs. Golashevsky's apartment. She found her lying in bed, weak and pale, barely able to move. The apartment was a mess, and it was clear that Mrs. Golashevsky had not been eating for days. Rachel called 911, and accompanied Mrs. Golashevsky to the hospital where she was found to have a colon cancer that was nearly obstructing her bowel and was slowly oozing blood.

The next morning Mrs. Golashevsky underwent surgery to remove the tumor. Unfortunately, at the time of surgery her entire abdominal cavity was found to be full of cancer. Malignant cells had spread everywhere, and virtually every organ surface was covered with thick tumor nodules.

Mrs. Golashevsky had tolerated her surgery remarkably well. She was awake, alert, sitting up in bed, and appeared to be recovering without difficulty. However, the serious problem of her very advanced cancer remained. This was the reason I had been called to see her.

I knocked softly on the door and heard a voice say, "Come in," before I entered the room. Upon entering, I saw a sweet and gentle-looking petite lady with curly gray hair. She was sitting up in bed with several pillows behind her. A nasogastric tube emerged from her left nostril and was hooked up to a suction apparatus on the wall. She looked very tired and very sad. Sitting on a chair close to the bed was a younger woman, about thirty-five years old.

"Good morning, Mrs. Golashevsky," I said, smiling at her. "I'm Dr. Geffen. Dr. Cooper, your surgeon, asked me to come and see you today. I'm pleased to meet you."

I offered Mrs. Golashevsky my hand, and we shook hands gently. Her hand was very small and warm. She looked at the other woman, who said something to her in Polish.

Mrs. Golashevsky then looked at me, and said, "Thank you," with a thick Polish accent.

We looked across the bed at each other, and even though she was only a few feet away, it seemed as if we were separated by a thousand miles. I realized that she had lived through events that I could only try to imagine—and now she was undergoing yet another tremendous challenge. She seemed so tired and lonely. I tried to silently embrace and reassure her with my eyes, and my thoughts: *It's okay, Mrs. Golashevsky. You don't have to be scared. I won't hurt you. I'm here to love and care for you, and to help in any way that I can.*

I turned to the other woman in the chair, and introduced myself again. "Hi, Dr. Geffen," she said. "My name is Rachel Kosala. I'm a friend of Mrs. Golashevsky, from the Polish American Club. Thank you for coming. She's a bit nervous right now, but I'm sure you can understand."

"Of course," I replied.

At that point I wanted to sit down and talk with them some more. Glancing around the room, I noticed that there were no other chairs. So I asked Mrs. Golashevsky if I could sit down beside her on the bed. She was staring at me intently, sizing me up. I smiled at her and waited to see if I would pass the test. Luckily I did. She slowly nodded and motioned to where she wanted me to sit.

I carefully sat down at the appointed place.

"How are you feeling today?" I began.

Before answering me, Mrs. Golashevsky turned to Rachel and spoke to her in Polish, and Rachel responded. Listening to them, I felt as if I had been transported to somewhere in Eastern Europe, in another time and place. I enjoyed the sound of their language. It reminded me of when I was a child, hearing Russian, Polish, Yiddish, and Hebrew spoken in my grandparents' home.

Finally, Mrs. Golashevsky looked at me and replied to my question. "I feel okay," she said in her thick accent.

"Do you have any pain?" I asked.

"No, thank God," she said.

"Do you feel nauseated?" I asked.

"No."

"Are you comfortable in your room?"

"Yes."

"Have you had any vomiting?"

"No."

"Any other problems?"

"No."

After asking a few more questions like these I felt reassured that she was not having any acute problems that needed to be addressed right away. I also felt that she was beginning to develop some trust in me, so I decided to try to go to the next level in our discussion.

"Mrs. Golashevsky," I asked gently, "do you understand why you are here in the hospital?"

She paused for a long time before answering, "Yes."

"Why?" I asked.

She exchanged a few words back and forth with Rachel before answering, "Because I have cancer."

"That's correct," I replied. "And do you understand why I am here to see you today?"

Once again she and Rachel spoke in Polish before she answered.

"Yes. Because you are a cancer doctor."

Another long pause. Then Mrs. Golashevsky spontaneously asked, "Can you help me, Doctor? I am so afraid."

"What are you afraid of?" I asked.

This time, she paused for a very, very long time.

"I am afraid that I am going to die."

I also paused, before asking, "What is it that makes you feel you are going to die?"

Mrs. Golashevsky again turned to Rachel, and they spoke together in Polish before she turned to me and said, "Because the cancer has spread throughout my abdomen. Dr. Cooper said it couldn't be cured with surgery. He said I needed to see you. When I asked him if you could cure me, he said he didn't know—but he didn't think so. So I am afraid I am going to die."

I took a deep breath and started to think about how to respond in the most sensitive and appropriate way. This was a tough situation. Colon cancer that has spread so extensively is generally incurable with any known means, particularly in someone as frail and weak as Mrs. Golashevsky. Fortunately many patients can have the quality of their life improved with chemotherapy treatments that are relatively mild and easy to tolerate. Some may even have their lives extended as well.

I explained all of this to Mrs. Golashevsky and asked if she was interested in talking further about some chemotherapy treatments that might help her.

I was surprised when she said no. And then, she began to sob uncontrollably.

I took her hand and tried to soothe her. After a minute or two she stopped crying, and I asked, "Why are you crying, Mrs. Golashevsky?"

"Because I am afraid to die."

"Then why don't you want treatment for your cancer? It might help you to live longer."

"I don't want any treatment for my cancer. I am all alone. My husband is gone, and I have no children. Why should I go through this? I have lived a good life, and have been blessed in many ways. But I am ready to go now. There is nothing to keep me here any longer."

I was impressed by her clarity, and by her honesty with herself and me. This is not such a common thing to see.

"Okay, Mrs. Golashevsky," I said. "I understand how you feel, and I can accept it if you are sure that is what you want. But I don't understand, then, why you were crying so."

"Because I am afraid to die," she said again.

"Please tell me," I said, "why are you so afraid to die?"

Once again she started to cry. This time she gave a long answer to my question in Polish, right through her tears.

Rachel translated for me: "Even though Mrs. Golashevsky feels she has had many blessings in her life, she has also suffered a great deal. She lived through so many deaths, and so many horrible things, especially during the war. She has terrifying images of death in her mind. She is terrified that when she dies she will suffer again. And she has seen so much suffering. How could she not be terrified?"

I looked at Mrs. Golashevsky. She was trembling with fear.

"Please tell her," I said to Rachel, "that she is not going to die right now. And when her time to die does come, she won't have to suffer. Tell her I will make sure she is comfortable."

Rachel translated and Mrs. Golashevsky seemed to understand. She calmed down, and we resumed talking about her current situation. At first everything went well, but soon she started to cry uncontrollably again.

I soon realized that I had to do something significant to shift her focus and her emotional state. The depth of her fear and her negative associations of death and dying were overwhelming her and dragging her deeper and deeper into despair. She kept on crying and sobbing, and was not responding to anything that Rachel or I said to her. But I knew I had to do something, *now*. I silently asked for some kind of inner guidance: *How could I help her? What could I possibly say or do that would be of help? How could I ease her pain and relieve her overwhelming fear?*

Then, in a flash, I remembered a beautiful story that I had once heard, and I thought, *This is it. This will work.*

I took a deep breath and looked at Mrs. Golashevsky, still crying and shaking before me.

"Mrs. Golashevsky," I said, "may I please ask you a question?"

She didn't hear me, so I repeated myself again, louder this time.

Mrs. Golashevsky continued crying, saying, "No. No. No."

I looked at Rachel, and pleaded with my eyes for her help.

"Katrina!" she shouted. "Katrina, listen! Dr. Geffen wants to ask you a question!"

Mrs. Golashevsky stopped crying for a moment and looked at me, still shivering in fear.

"What?" she asked.

"Mrs. Golashevsky, please tell me something. It is very important. I need to know. When you were a very little girl, *did you go to school*?"

I watched the question enter Mrs. Golashevsky's consciousness, and I saw it start to work its magic. At first she looked confused, with an expression on her face that seemed to say, *Of course I went to school. Why in the world are you asking me that? What on earth does that have to do with anything that is happening right now?*

This is exactly what I had hoped would happen. She was no longer thinking of her horrible fears about death.

"Yes," she finally replied.

"Good," I answered. "Now I need to know something else. This is also very important. When you were a little girl, *did you like going to school*?"

I continued to watch her carefully as she thought about my question. I could see from the expression on her face that she was beginning to call up new images in her mind, images of when she was a little girl, before the war.

Slowly, as the expression on her face continued to change, I could tell we were on the right track. After a moment or two, she started to smile, tentatively.

"Great," I said. "Now, this is really important. I really need to know, so I will ask you again. When you were a little girl, *did you like going to school*?"

Now, Mrs. Golashevsky broke into a smile, and nodding her head, said, "Oh yes. Very much."

Rachel and I both breathed a big sigh of relief. It was clear that her focus had now changed significantly. The tension in the room lifted, and Mrs. Golashevsky stopped shaking and trembling altogether.

I decided to go further.

"Great. Now, Mrs. Golashevsky, I have another question. When you were a little girl, did you ever get a new pair of shoes?"

Once again Mrs. Golashevsky looked puzzled by my question. Rachel and I sighed as her eyes seemed to light up, and she nodded yes.

"Did you ever get a new pair of shoes that you *really loved a lot*?"

"Yes," she answered.

"Can you remember what they looked like?"

"Oh yes," she said.

"How old were you then?" I asked.

After a few moments she said, "Ten years old."

Mrs. Golashevsky's eyes were now starting to actually sparkle. We could see she was *there,* reliving the memory of being ten years old and getting her new pair of shoes.

"What color were they?" I asked.

"They were black," she said, "and very shiny. My father bought them for me. They were my birthday present. He worked so hard to get them."

"Do you remember the first time you wore them?" I asked.

"Yes, I remember it very well. It was the first day of school."

"Great," I said. "Do you remember how it felt wearing them to school for the first time?"

"Oh yes. I loved them, and felt so proud wearing them."

"Let me ask you another question. Were your shoes a bit tight and stiff the first time you wore them?"

"Yes."

"Did they hurt to walk around in when they were new?" I asked.

"Actually, yes," she replied.

"I can imagine that very well. Very often that is how shoes feel when they are new, when you wear them for the first time. Now, Mrs. Golashevsky, I want to ask you another question. On that first day when you wore your new shoes to school, did you wear them all day?"

She closed her eyes and remembered the day. "Yes," she said.

"And can you remember walking home in your new shoes?"

"Yes."

"And can you remember how your feet felt when you finally got home from school that day?"

"Yes."

"How did they feel?"

"They hurt. *A lot.* By the time I got home my feet were really hurting."

"Exactly," I said. "Now I want to ask you one last question, Mrs. Golashevsky. Do you remember when you finally got home, and you took your shoes off? Do you remember that moment? Do you remember how it felt?"

She closed her eyes once again and went back in time to that moment as a ten-year-old-girl, taking off her stiff and tight-fitting shoes. Then she started to smile and opened her eyes to look at me.

"Yes," she said, "I remember."

"How did it feel?" I asked.

"Ahhh," she said, "it felt so good. It felt *wonderful.*"

"That's right, Mrs. Golashevsky," I said. "I can imagine how good it felt. And guess what?" I asked.

"What?" she replied.

"Dying is just like that. *Dying is like taking off a pair of tight-fitting shoes.* It doesn't hurt at all. It is completely safe. And there is nothing to be afraid of."

Mrs. Golashevsky smiled back at me, and her eyes sparkled and filled with tears. She got it. She understood. She nodded, and said in Polish, "I see. I see."

Soon we finished up our visit for the day. We had covered a lot of ground, and she needed to rest. I said good-bye and promised to return the next morning. We talked more each day while she remained in the hospital. During this time she continued to say no whenever I asked her if she wanted to consider receiving any further treatment. After about a week she left the hospital and returned to her apartment, feeling much stronger.

A few days later she came to my office to talk further about her situation. Rachel, who brought her in, had many new questions. Mrs. Golashevsky's abdomen was starting to fill up with fluid, and we talked about things that could be done to help relieve this. However, Mrs. Golashevsky was still not interested in treatment. She wasn't having any pain or discomfort and didn't want the fluid drained off. And she definitely didn't want chemotherapy.

What she really wanted was to see me every week, and have a chance to talk.

And so, we did. Each week she would come in for a visit, and I would examine her carefully and review how she was feeling. During these visits we talked about everything, including her childhood, and so many of the things she had lived through. We would also occasionally talk about that beautiful pair of tight-fitting shoes that she loved so much, which had now developed a new and even deeper meaning for her. Little by little, even though her body was slowly dying, inside she seemed more alive. And little by little, each time we talked, her fear of death diminished.

After a while Mrs. Golashevsky decided that she would allow me to drain off the fluid in her abdomen, which had started to make her uncomfortable. This provided her great, and instant, relief. She was amazed at how dramatic the effects were. But she still refused to consider undergoing treatment with chemotherapy to try to extend her life.

The fluid soon reaccumulated in her abdomen, and she needed to have the procedure performed weekly. Initially, she didn't mind at all. It got her out of the house and kept her going.

During this time we openly discussed the fact that her cancer was inevitably going to take her life. I asked Mrs. Golashevsky if she wanted to be at home when her time came to die, or if she would prefer to be in the hospital. By now she was no longer terrified of dying and was quite clear about her wishes. "I want to be at home," she said without hesitation. "And I want Rachel to be there with me." I asked Rachel if she agreed, and she said, "Yes, of course." So Mrs. Golashevsky was enrolled into the hospice program, and all the appropriate arrangements were made so she could be at home, safely and comfortably, until the end.

A week later the swelling in her abdomen increased dramatically—much more than on previous occasions. She started to have severe pain and felt much weaker than before. Moving around now required great effort. Her interest in eating, or in doing anything at all, faded and disappeared. But she insisted that Rachel bring her to see me one last time.

She arrived in a wheelchair, a blanket wrapped around her legs, looking so thin and frail. Her eyes were tired but also filled with determination to see me. While examining her I felt heartsick, because there was no question that her cancer had now reached a very advanced stage. When I explained this to her and Rachel, Mrs. Golashevsky softly asked, "Am I going to die now, Dr. Geffen?"

"Probably not today, Mrs. Golashevsky, but I'm afraid probably soon," I replied. We reviewed everything one last time, and she confirmed her feeling that she had made the right choice for her. She also confirmed that she didn't want any more treatments of any kind, and that she was now truly ready to let go. She had insisted on coming in today only because she wanted to hear from me directly what she intuitively knew was happening. And she wanted to say good-bye, in person.

We hugged each other, then sat quietly together for a few minutes. We spoke again about her life, and how we had met in the hospital all those weeks before. We talked about all she had been through, including her impending death, which no longer terrified her. And we talked once more about her childhood, and that pair of beautiful shoes she loved so much.

Finally, it was time to go. I promised her again that I would make sure she was comfortable all the way till the end, and that she would have no pain. We laughed, cried, and hugged once more, and said good-bye one last time.

As she and Rachel left, my heart was sad, but also filled with love and appreciation for her. What a beautiful, courageous soul Mrs. Golashevsky was. I knew I was blessed to have met her.

Two weeks later I received a letter from Rachel.

> *Dear Dr. Geffen,*
>   *Last Tuesday morning, at 2:30 A.M., Mrs. Golashevsky took off her shoes, as I held her hand.*
>   *Thank you for everything.*
>   *With love,*
>   *Rachel*

10

LEVEL SEVEN:
THE NATURE OF SPIRIT

SILENCE IS THE ABSOLUTE POISE OR BALANCE OF
BODY, MIND AND SPIRIT. THE MAN WHO
PERCEIVES HIS SELFHOOD IS EVER CALM AND
UNSHAKEN BY THE STORMS OF EXISTENCE.
                                    —OHIYESA (1858–1939)

I AM THE SELF THAT RESIDES IN THE HEART OF
ALL BEINGS.
                                    —BHAGAVAD GITA

WHATEVER BE THE MEANS ADOPTED, YOU MUST AT
LAST RETURN TO THE SELF. SO WHY NOT ABIDE IN
THE SELF HERE AND NOW?
       —BHAGAVAN SRI RAMANA MAHARSHI (1879–1950)

Who are you?
       It's a deceptively simple question. Are you your body? Are
you your mind? Are you the feelings in your heart? If you *have*
a body, mind, and heart, can you also *be* those things? And if you are not
those things, then what are you?

So far, we've given our attention to the physical, mental, and emotional aspects of our ourselves. Now, in this seventh level, we will open
our eyes to a whole new dimension of being—the dimension of spirit.

This dimension is different in a number of important ways. It is also vitally important in the journey through cancer.

Most of us, out of necessity, live our lives on the surface of things. We're like the navigators of ships; our greatest concern is to get from the point of departure to our destination, often as quickly as possible. Needless to say, the waters can get choppy—and rarely more so than after a diagnosis of cancer.

At such a time, our primary concern is certainly the immediate clinical issues—the high winds and waves, if you will. But it is a mistake to focus on these issues exclusively. The journey through cancer is a time when it is vitally important to look beneath the surface, into the vast depths that are untouched by even the greatest and most turbulent waves.

This exploration is not simply a digression or distraction from the "real world." The profound serenity that underlies our everyday experience is, in a sense, the *real* real world.

When your attention is directed toward the dimension of spirit, even for just a few minutes each day, your entire experience of life can be transformed. Just a glimpse of this reality can change everything. It is as if someone who had been born and raised in an enclosed room is one day shown a window on the world. All it takes is one glance, one breath of fresh air, one glimpse of the larger environment, and their understanding of reality is expanded exponentially. From that moment on, life will never be the same.

By discovering the realm of spirit, many people with cancer have this very experience. Their illness has isolated them, both physically and emotionally, from the world at large. Cancer and its treatments can be so overwhelming that the possibility of another reality may seem inconceivable. But another reality does exist.

The window to this reality opens when you sit quietly, allow the mind to calm down, and begin to look within your own self. There you will find a world that can never be fully reached through thought, effort, or activity of any kind—a gentle, silent awareness and presence of love and joy that lies within the heart of every being. This reality is always present. It is that aspect of ourselves that is timeless, dimensionless, and untouched by any circumstance—including illness, disease, cancer, and even death.

When patients and their family members are in touch with this part of themselves, their experience of the journey through cancer can change in extraordinary ways. The process is greatly enhanced when some time is taken each day to shift awareness away from the all-consuming drama of the physical body, and the emotional storms that are often a part of the drama. By entering the dimension of being that is untouched by events in the mental, emotional, and physical realms, the peaks and valleys of the journey are softened. A genuine sense of peace and serenity can appear—even in the midst of the fiercest storms—that is of tremendous benefit to everyone.

By nurturing an ongoing awareness of the deepest level of self, patients gain direct access to the most profound source of the love and joy we all seek. Though at times it may be difficult to grasp, the realm of spirit is actually the source of everything that cancer patients and their families really want. This includes not only love and joy but physical healing as well. Although consciously allowing your awareness to abide in the realm of spirit on a regular basis is not a guarantee that physical healing will occur, I deeply believe that it improves the chances, perhaps significantly.

Incorporating a spiritual dimension into the practice of medicine brings joy and fulfillment not only to patients but to doctors, nurses, and all other members of the health care team as well. Something profoundly healing and uplifting occurs in acknowledging the aspect of our work that reaches beyond the physical realm. When we take the time to honor and care for the spiritual dimension of life that we all share—no matter what role we happen to be playing in the journey—everyone gains.

This is an extremely important point, because a new vision of medicine that embraces all the dimensions of who we are as human beings must include awareness of the consciousness and intentions of the caregivers. We can't give what we don't have. We cannot help people heal as deeply as we want, or as deeply as they want, unless *we ourselves* are healed.

ENTERING THE REALM OF SPIRIT

Finding our spiritual essence is an intimate process of self-discovery. Most often it takes place through time spent in silence, in meditation and prayer, in nature, and in communion with family, friends, loved ones, and other patients.

Drugs and radiation may kill cancer cells, but they don't make a human being healthy or joyful. That power comes from spirit. In addition—and my words are chosen carefully here—if so-called spontaneous recoveries or remissions do occur, they must ultimately come along this pathway. They will enter your body through your soul—yet, remarkably, even the soul is not the deepest truth of who you are.

The soul is the first ripple of individuality on a vast ocean of pure awareness that underlies everything in existence. That ripple eventually grows into a solid wave, until the physical body comes into being. If we wish to find the true origin of the physical body, we must go all the way to the ultimate source. Stopping at the wave is not going all the way home.

"You are not the wave," said Ramana Maharshi, one of India's greatest and most revered sages. "You are the ocean."

Indeed, who we all truly are is the vast and timeless ocean of awareness out of which every being, and in fact all of creation, arises and eventually falls away. By recognizing your real identity as the ocean rather than the wave—regardless of how healthy, diseased, powerful, or powerless the wave may appear—you can find freedom not only from cancer, but even from birth and death. That is the ultimate message of this book.

ASKING THE ULTIMATE QUESTIONS

In our daily lives, we view ourselves as separate beings, or as separate waves, existing independently from one another. Our common perception is that we are limited in time and space by our physical bodies, our personal histories, our worldly identities, and our unique memories, hopes, fears, and desires. In fact, we tend to identify *completely* with these aspects of ourselves.

For both classical Buddhism and the Vedic traditions of India, however, the experience of an independent self is an illusion. Clinging to the false idea of an independent self is regarded as the fundamental cause of the suffering, illness, disease, and death that human beings experience over and over again. This attachment, and all the suffering that goes with it, arises from a basic misunderstanding about our true nature.

On a relative level, we do experience ourselves as solid, separate physical beings. But at a deeper level of reality this is a misperception. When the illusion of our separateness is dispelled, the interconnectedness of everything is clearly seen and understood. The level of reality at which this interconnectedness exists is the "ocean of awareness" referred to earlier. Throughout history, this reality has been given many different names by the great spiritual traditions of the world. In Buddhism, it is called *Shunyata,* or "emptiness." In the Vedic tradition it is called *Brahman,* or the Self. This transcendent reality does not exist at some point lights years away. It exists within *each of us.* At the ultimate level, it is the deepest truth of who we really are.

In Sanskrit, one of the most powerful expressions of this truth is *Aham Brahmasmi,* or "I am That." And That which I am—and which we *all* are—is absolutely still, immaculate, and pure. It is beyond conception, beyond birth and death, and beyond illness of any kind.

Thousands of years ago, the sages of ancient India saw and understood the unity, the oneness, underlying all of creation and recognized that we are not separate from that oneness in any way. Twenty-five hundred years ago, Buddha also saw and understood the fundamental illusion of the separate self. Since then, mystics and saints from all the world's religious and spiritual traditions have proclaimed this same truth. Remarkably, in the twentieth century, Albert Einstein arrived at the same conclusion, which he described this way:

> *A human being is part of the whole, called by us the universe, a part limited in time and space. He experiences himself, his thoughts, and feelings as something separated from the rest…a kind of optical delusion of his consciousness.*

In facing cancer, and in directly confronting the very real possibility of death, patients and their family members have a pressing need and opportunity to examine this question of who we all really are. Few people ever do this without the imperative of a serious illness. But cancer can bring the question into sharp focus, often like nothing else. Finding the most enlightened answer is the ultimate reward of the journey through cancer, and the journey through life.

WHAT IS THE ULTIMATE CAUSE OF CANCER?

Discussion of ultimate realities offers an opportunity to address this important and mysterious question. As with most fundamental questions, the answer depends on the point of view of the questioner.

If you perceive your existence in terms of a physical body that is born and dies, whose consciousness is wholly dependent upon brain activity and function, your viewpoint is consistent with the current biomolecular model of medicine. In that worldview, cancer is caused by oncogene or tumor-suppressor gene derangements. Those derangements in turn are caused by physical events occurring in the external world, initiated by various toxins or by events in the internal world, precipitated by hormonal or other biochemical changes in the body or by inherited genetic predispositions. This is the cause of cancer on the relative level of existence.

Another point of view might find the cause of cancer in God, or even the devil. Perhaps there is an omnipotent being who works in inscrutable ways—to punish, reward, or test the faith and endurance of individuals. In this view, the cause of disease is often related to the concepts of right and wrong, good and evil, or virtue and sin.

An atheistic or existential philosophy might see cancer, and life itself, as a completely random event that is entirely without meaning. For individuals who hold this point of view, there is no more "meaning" in cancer than there is in the flip of a coin.

Finally, there is what I consider to be the enlightened view, in which the universe is recognized to be an emanation of our own consciousness. In this view, nothing exists independently of our own perception, understanding, and ultimate intention. Despite the experience of our senses, despite appearances to the contrary, in truth we are not separate from anything in the universe at all. Who we are is indeed the pure ocean of awareness out of which everything arises and falls away again.

The ultimate serenity of spirit that patients discover in Level Seven is intimately linked with this understanding and direct experience of our oneness with all of existence. An additional aspect of this involves the recognition that who we are at the deepest level is also never truly touched by the storms of existence.

When there is a storm at sea, at the very bottom of the ocean there is stillness. No matter how turbulent the waves appear on the surface, the bottom of the ocean remains still, silent, and untouched. In a similar way, we are not the images that appear and disappear in life. In fact, our awareness itself is the screen onto which the images of life are projected. Regardless of the content of those images—whether they contain fire, earthquakes, hurricanes, or even nuclear explosions—the screen itself is always unaffected. Thus also with the "movie" of cancer. The drama feels and appears very real, but in every moment, at the deepest level of reality, the timeless, dimensionless, inner Self is untouched by it.

It is important to remember that I am in no way suggesting that we ignore the outer world of appearances in which we abide—the domain of *doing*—which includes the worlds of sensory experience, everyday life, and comprehensive cancer treatment. I firmly advocate doing everything possible to help people heal and transform physically, mentally, and emotionally. But in Level Seven of this program another possibility is revealed. That possibility is the invitation to acknowledge and embrace the other domain of existence—the domain of *being*—that exists simultaneously with the domain of doing. This domain of being is the doorway to ultimate freedom and to the ultimate healing journey. For this doorway leads to the recognition of our true nature, the true Self, the truth of who we all are—beyond what can be seen and known, beyond name and form, and beyond time and space. This truth of who we all are is not separate in any way from God, the cosmos, and all that exists.

How is this related to the cause of cancer? As long as you regard yourself as an individual being who is isolated and separate from others, and from creation itself, you will experience yourself as being subject to the laws of nature, physics, and biology.

You may also experience yourself as an independent soul on a journey toward enlightenment. According to Eastern philosophy, this soul will reincarnate through many lifetimes and will experience events in each life according to its own prior actions. There is no God "out there" who is rewarding you or punishing you. Rather, each of us experiences the results of our own actions, both positive and negative, which is called *karma*.

This is not to say that getting cancer is a punishment for behavior in past lives. It just means that the seed of this experience has been planted in some way by ourselves—by our own thoughts, feelings, and actions—at some point in the past. Perhaps it is a lesson that you yourself have chosen to learn, or a dimension of human experience that you have chosen to understand. The individual soul wants to grow, to learn and expand, and ultimately to discover and experience the fullness of itself. The wave wants to experience itself as a wave, with all its ups and downs, before falling back into the ocean and remembering its true identity.

Karma is unrelated to punishment, or reward. It is simply the law of cause and effect. If you water a plant, it will grow. If you don't, it will die—with no guilt or judgment involved. Ultimately, since we are not separate from all that exists, there are no "events" that occur "out there" without our involvement; indeed without our active participation on some level, no matter how remote that level may appear.

From this perspective, one could definitely say that we all choose the events of our lives because we want to learn and grow—and sometimes, we learn and grow best from painful and difficult experiences. You have not chosen them to punish yourself, but to gain what's needed to move forward on your journey.

It is impossible for ordinary people to really know *why* something happens to one person and not to another. Only truly enlightened people can comprehend why things happen as they do. But knowing *why* is not the most important thing. "Why me?" is a disempowering question. The better questions are:

What can I do now to make the most of this experience?

How can I learn and grow best from my illness?

How can I use this experience to discover and fulfill the purpose of my life?

How can I use this journey through cancer to discover my own true Self?

11

CONCLUSION

SOMEDAY, AFTER WE HAVE MASTERED THE WINDS,
THE WAVES, THE TIDE AND GRAVITY, WE SHALL
HARNESS FOR GOD THE ENERGIES OF LOVE. AND
THEN, FOR THE SECOND TIME IN THE HISTORY OF
THE WORLD, MAN WILL HAVE DISCOVERED FIRE.

—TEILHARD DE CHARDIN

I remember one of the final conversations I had with my father, just a few short weeks after we took that taxi ride together through Central Park. This time we were in his hospital room, and he was approaching the very end of his life.

We were sitting together, in silence. Drinking together, from the river of silence.

Without speaking, we were appreciating all that we had lived and shared in this life.

Without speaking, we were treasuring our last hours and moments together, and acknowledging how much we were going to miss each other.

And without speaking, we were saying our final good-byes.

Then, suddenly, I felt a deep and powerful presence of energy in the room. I looked up and saw my father beaming, grinning from ear to ear. He looked back at me, and his face was filled with a quiet, peaceful radiance. The room was very still, and I was aware of sunlight streaming in the window.

Quietly, I said, "Sid, what's going on?"

"Jeremy," he answered, "I'm so happy. I'm so happy. I'm so happy."

His words startled me, because here was my father, a relatively young man—only sixty-one years old—lying in a hospital bed, dying. His lungs were filled with metastatic gastric cancer, and his belly was filled with gastric cancer and ascites. He was barely able to move without pain. Barely able to breathe without oxygen. And yet, here he was, saying *he's so happy.*

"How can this be?" I asked. "Please tell me."

"I'm so happy," he replied, "because now I really understand. It's all so clear. We are not our positions, and we are not our possessions. *All we are is love. All that exists is love. And, all that matters is love.* And in seeing this, I'm so happy."

For me, the kind of awareness that my father had in that moment represents the true power and significance of the vision of medicine and healing that we have explored in this book. This is a vision that honors and cares for the body, mind, heart, and spirit of all beings with equal skill, strength, and integrity. It is a vision that honors all paths of healing, from every culture in the world, in a spirit of humility, open-mindedness, and respect. And it is a vision that recognizes the dimension of who we are as humans, beyond all appearances, that is the source of the love, joy, and fulfillment that we all seek.

There is no question in my mind that as our understanding deepens of how all the dimensions of ourselves are interwoven, and how different approaches to medicine can likewise be interwoven into a tapestry of stunning beauty and power, we will discover ways of healing ourselves and one another we could never have imagined before.

And as we proceed further on this amazing journey that we are all taking, we will learn something else. As we continue our adventure through the ever-changing and extraordinary realms of medicine and healing, through the domain of doing into the domain of being, from action into stillness, from speech into silence, we will appreciate even more the great mystery of how the body, mind, heart, and spirit are not only interwoven but indeed are *one and the same.* Here, we will ultimately discover our true nature as human beings and the essence of *who we really are.* In doing so, I am certain, we will come to understand the true meaning of love, the power of love, and the meaning of life itself.

ACKNOWLEDGMENTS

The Journey Through Cancer has been as much a labor of love and the heart as it has been an effort of the mind and intellect. One of the greatest joys in completing it is the opportunity to publicly thank all those individuals who have made such an important contribution to my life over so many years.

Thus, I wish to say "Thank You," from my heart,

To my grandfather, David Geffen, who demonstrated honor, wisdom, humility, and integrity in all aspects of his life, and who inspired in me a deep love of learning, education, knowledge, and contribution;

To my father, Sidney Geffen, who showed me the example of a man who always followed his dream, even in the face of incredible pressure, and who always saw the humor and irony of life;

To my uncle, Merwin Geffen, MD, for his love, guidance, and never-ending support and encouragement;

To my mother, Dita Geffen, who showed me that a mother's love truly never dies; and to my dear sisters: Talia Cohen, Danah Geffen, and Amara Geffen, who have loved and supported me through all the years;

To my editor, Ann Patty, at Crown, for her courage, faith, support, and determination to get the message of *The Journey Through Cancer* out to the millions of people in the world who we both sincerely hope and believe will benefit from it;

To my agent, Kris Dahl, at ICM, for seeing and understanding the vision of *The Journey Through Cancer,* for her support and encouragement, and for taking a chance with an unknown writer;

To Mitch Sisskind, for his invaluable contributions in preparing the manuscript, for his friendship and support, and for our innumerable, heartfelt dialogues about this book and so many of the deep issues of life;

To Michael Rudell, Esq., Jason Baruch, Esq., and Neil Rosini, Esq., for their wise, skillful, and deeply appreciated guidance and support throughout the planning and development of *The Journey Through Cancer*;

To Dr. Paul Bass, the world's greatest coach, for his love, faith, confidence and support, for teaching me so much, and for standing with me through so many tough times;

To the entire staff of the Geffen Cancer Center and Research Institute—including Al Boileau, MT, Trish Garey, Richard Hocking, Shirley Ketchpaw, Mimi Koerner, Jennifer Lang, LPN, Darlene Lieffort, CLNI, Charlotte Millspaugh, LCSW, Russell Shoemaker, Linda Smith, Hidi St. Peter, Connie Tarasavage, LPN, LMT, Donna Terrill, BSN, OCN, CRNI, and Sandra Woods—for their incredible hard work, sacrifice, courage, and faith in helping to fulfill our vision, and for the meticulous, impeccable, and loving care that they consistently give to all of our patients and their family members;

To Debra Dickerson, CLNI, who was with me at the birth of the Cancer Center and the Seven-Level Program, for her years of unwavering love, support, hard work, encouragement, and dedication to our vision;

To Rita Rosko, for all her meals, laughter, and hugs, for caring for me with such love and devotion over the years, and for always being there;

To Julie and S. T. Forgione, Surja Jessup, Sonni Kane, Mary Ann Cooke, Sue Lewis, Bill Servis, and Melissa Webster for their extraordinary friendship and unwavering support;

To David Simon, MD, and Deepak Chopra, MD, for their contributions to bringing the light of knowledge and wisdom into the world, for their friendship, and for their confidence and support;

To Bob Harris, CPA, Ross Cotherman, CPA, Cheri Jones, CPA, John Moore, Esq., Brad Rossway, Esq., Barry Oberholtzer, and Laura Koenigsaecker, for believing in me and the vision of the Geffen Cancer Center and Research Institute, and for all their help and support;

To Jana Pallis, Lexie Brockway Potamkin, Kathy Zavada, Bev and Bruce Gordon, Anna Triebel Thome, Brandon Bays, Debra Angeletti, Bill and Penny George, Carole Abrahams, Debra Frasier, Jenny and Randy Gilford, Staton and Tabitha Grant, Lorraine and Lou Blankenmeier, Cristina Santaella, Amy Lee, Michael Sautman, Allen Keller, MD, Howard Frumkin, MD, Danny and Stacey Hersh, Shana Stanberry, ScD, Penelope Young, LCSW, Michael Spatuzzi, David Cornsweet, PhD, Susan Osborn, Paul Winter, Diane Agnello, Joan Brady, Claire O'Daniel, Michael Stillwater, Hector Moré, Esq., Ben Newman, Esq., David Illig, PhD, Sandy Sela-Smith, Sal Tarsitano, Jack, Sally and Shyamala Ruane, Yashoda Hutner, Ananda Devi, Neeraja Tronca, Gopal Verhague, and Mira Decoux, for their love, support, and friendship;

To Deb Hinz, and Anthony and Becky Robbins, for their very special love, support, and inspiration;

To John Suen, MD, for his amazing support, friendship, and encouragement during some of the most extraordinary and challenging years of our lives;

To my colleagues and friends at Indian River Memorial Hospital, for their friendship and support over the years we have worked together;

To Robert Compton, Esq., Eddi Winter, Jana Barile, Jerry Swanson, Gage Gwyn, ARNP, and Lora Grabach, for their important and deeply appreciated contributions in the early years of the Cancer Center;

To Ash Andon, for his unwavering love, faith, confidence, and support;

To Philip Lee, MD, Frank Valone, MD, Michael Weiner, MD, Alan Venook, MD, Stephen Wasserman, MD, and Alvin Friedman-Kien, MD, for their support and encouragement during my years in academic medicine;

To all the doctors, nurses, and caregivers who work so hard and give so much, through long days and even longer nights, caring for the sick and weary, who have taught me so much and whose lives are an example for the world;

To Shirley Green and Thomas Byrom, who walked the journey through cancer with incredible grace, humility, compassion, dignity, and love for everyone around them;

And finally…

To Neem Karoli Baba, for wrapping me in his blanket when I was so young, and for keeping me there always;

To Ma Jaya Sati Bhagavati, for her years of love and support, for her radiant, shining example of passionate love and devotion to God and humanity, for showing me the River…and teaching me to swim;

and to H. W. L. Poonja, known to so many as Papaji, for his supreme gifts of the Ocean, and of Silence. I bow in gratitude.

SOURCES AND
SELECTED REFERENCES

CHAPTER 1: WHAT IS THE PURPOSE OF MEDICINE?

Clifford, Terry. *Tibetan Buddhist Medicine and Psychiatry: The Diamond Healing.* York Beach, ME: Samuel Weiser, Inc. 1984.

Devrode G. On a practitioner's "being" as the true healing agent. *Advances in Mind-Body Medicine.* 1999;15:134–136.

Dossey L. Do religion and spirituality matter in health? A response to the recent article in *The Lancet.* [special commentary] *Alternative Therapies in Health and Medicine.* 1999;5(3):16–18.

Godman, David, ed. *Be as You Are: The Teachings of Sri Ramana Maharshi.* London: Arkana Books. 1991.

Kahn DL and Steeves RH. Spiritual well-being: a review of the research literature. *Quality of Life—A Nursing Challenge.* 1993;2(3):60–64.

Lintz KC, Penson RT, Chabner BA, and Lynch TJ. A staff dialogue on caring for an intensely spiritual patient: psychosocial issues faced by patients, their families, and caregivers. *The Oncologist.* 1998;3:439–445.

Passik SD, Dugan W, McDonald MV, et al. Oncologists' recognition of depression in their patients with cancer. *Journal of Clinical Oncology.* 1998;16(4):1594–1600.

Sloan RP, Bagiella E, and Powell T. Religion, spirituality, and medicine. *The Lancet.* 1999;353(9153):664–667.

Voljc B. On the spirituality of the doctor-patient relationship. *Annals of the New York Academy of Science.* 1997;809:80–82.

CHAPTER 2: BEVERLY IS EVERY ONE OF US

Brown ML. Special Report: The national economic burden of cancer: an update. *Journal of the National Cancer Institute.* 1990;82:1811–1814.

Calabresi P, Antman KH, Bettinghaus EP, et al. Cancer at a crossroads: A report to Congress for the nation. Subcommittee to Evaluate the National Cancer Program. National Cancer Advisory Board. National Cancer Institute. 1994.

Cassileth BR and Chapman CC. Alternative and Complementary Cancer Therapies. *Cancer.* 1996;77(6):1026–1034.

Cassileth BR, Lusk EJ, Strouse TB, and Bodebheimer BJ. Contemporary unorthodox treatments in cancer medicine: a study of patients, treatments and practitioners. *Annals of Internal Medicine.* 1984;101(1):105–112.

Downer SM, Cody MM, McCluskay P, et al. Pursuit and practice of complementary therapies by cancer patients receiving conventional treatment. *British Medical Journal.* 1994;309:86–89.

Eisenberg DM, Kessler RC, Foster C, et al. Unconventional medicine in the United States: prevalence, costs, and patterns of use. *New England Journal of Medicine.* 1993;328(4):246–252.

Eisenberg DM, Davis RB, Ettner SL, et al. Trends in alternative medicine use in the United States, 1990–1997: results of a follow-up national survey. *Journal of the American Medical Association.* 1998;280(18):1569–1575.

Ernst E and Cassileth BR. The prevalence of complementary/alternative medicine in cancer: a systematic review. *Cancer.* 1998;83(4):777–782.

Feuer EJ. Lifetime probability of cancer. *Journal of the National Cancer Institute.* 1997;89(4):279.

Fisher B, Dignam J, Wolmark N, et al. Tamoxifen and chemotherapy for lymph node–negative, estrogen receptor–positive breast cancer. *Journal of the National Cancer Institute.* 1997;89(22):1673–1682.

Fisher B, Dignam J, Wolmark N, et al. Tamoxifen in treatment of intraductal breast cancer: National Surgical Adjuvant Breast and Bowel Project B-24 randomized controlled trial. *The Lancet.* 1999;353:1993–2000.

Fraumeni JF, Devesa SS, Hoover RN, and Kinlen LJ. Epidemiology of cancer. In: DeVita VT, Hellman S, Rosenberg SA, eds. *Cancer: principles and practice of oncology.* [4th edition] Philadelphia: J. B. Lippincott Co. 1993:150–159.

Haas GP and Sakr WA. Epidemiology of prostate cancer. *CA: A Cancer Journal for Clinicians.* 1997;47(5):273–287.

Jacobsen SJ, Katusic SK, Bergstralh MS, et al. Incidence of prostate cancer diagnosis in the eras before and after serum prostate-specific antigen testing. *Journal of the American Medical Association.* 1995;274(18):1445–1449.

King SE and Schottenfeld D. The "epidemic" of breast cancer in the U.S.—determining the factors. *Oncology.* 1996;10(4):453–462.

Landis SH, Murray T, Bolden S, and Wingo PA. Cancer Statistics, 1999. *CA: A Cancer Journal for Clinicians.* 1999;49(1):8–31.

Lerner IJ and Kennedy BJ. The prevalence of questionable methods of cancer treatment in the United States. *CA: A Cancer Journal for Clinicians.* 1992;42(3):181–191.

McGinnis LS. Alternative therapies, 1990. *Cancer*. 1991;67(6)supp:1788–1792.

Parker SL, Tong T, Bolden S, and Wingo PA. Cancer Statistics, 1996. *CA: A Cancer Journal for Clinicians*. 1996;46(1):5–27.

Risberg T, Lund E, Wist E, et al. Cancer patients use of non-proven therapy: a 5-year follow-up study. *Journal of Clinical Oncology*. 1998;16(1):6–12.

Schuette HL, Tucker TC, Brown ML, et al. The costs of cancer care in the United States: implications for action. *Oncology*. 1995;9(11)supp:19–22.

Stat Bite: Cancer incidence trends in U.S. women. *Journal of the National Cancer Institute*. 1996;88(24):806.

Stat Bite: Cancer incidence trends in U.S. men. *Journal of the National Cancer Institute*. 1997;89(1):14.

VandeCreek L, Rogers E, and Lester J. Use of alternative therapies among breast cancer outpatients compared with the general population. *Alternative Therapies in Health and Medicine*. 1999;5(1):71–76.

CHAPTER 3: THE BASICS

Baselga J, Norton L, Albanell J, et al. Recombinant humanized anti-HER2 antibody (Herceptin) enhances the antitumor activity of paclitaxel and doxorubicin against HER2/neu overexpressing human breast cancer xenografts. *Cancer Research*. 1998;58(13):2825–2831.

Baselga J, Tripathy D, Mendelsohn J, et al. Phase II study of weekly intravenous recombinant humanized anti-p185^{HER2} monoclonal antibody in patients with HER2/*neu*-overexpressing metastatic breast cancer. *Journal of Clinical Oncology*. 1996;14(3):737–744.

Bonadonna G, Valagussa P, Moliterni A, et al. Adjuvant cyclophosphamide, methotrexate, and fluorouracil in node-positive breast cancer: the results of 20 years of follow-up. *New England Journal of Medicine*. 1995;332(14):901–906.

Bishop JM. Molecular themes in oncogenesis. *Cell*. 1991;64:23–38.

Bridge JA, Schwartz HS, and Neff JR. Bone sarcomas. In: Abeloff MD, Armitage JO, Lichter AS, and Niederhuber JE, eds. *Clinical Oncology*. New York: Churchill Livingstone. 1995:1715–1797.

Brinton LA and Hoover RN. Epidemiology of gynecologic cancers. In: *Principles and Practice of Gynecologic Oncology*. Hoskins WJ, Perez CA, and Young R, eds. [2nd edition] Philadelphia: Lippincott-Raven. 1997:3–29.

Carney DN. New agents in the management of advanced non–small cell lung cancer. *Seminars in Oncology*. 1998;25(4)supplement9:83–88.

Chang F, Syrjanen S, and Syrjanen K. Implications of the *p53* tumor-suppressor gene in clinical oncology. *Journal of Clinical Oncology*. 1995;13(4):1009–1022.

Collins FS, Patrinos A, Jordan E, et al. New goals for the U.S. Human Genome Project: 1998–2003. *Science*. 1998;282:682–689.

Damron TA and Pritchard DJ. Current combined treatment of high-grade osteosarcomas. *Oncology.* 1995;9(4):327–343.

Davis TA, White CA, Grillo-López AJ, et al. Single-agent monoclonal antibody efficacy in bulky non-Hodgkin's lymphoma: results of a phase II trial of rituximab. *Journal of Clinical Oncology.* 1999;17(6):1851–1857.

Denmeade SR and Isaacs JT. Programmed cell death (apoptosis) and cancer chemotherapy. *Cancer Control.* 1996;3(4):303–309.

Deisseroth A, Guo D, Wang T, et al. Molecular therapy for cancer. *The Cancer Journal.* 1998;4,supplement1:5–7.

Dranoff G. Cancer gene therapy: connecting basic research with clinical inquiry. *Journal of Clinical Oncology.* 1998;16(7):2548–2556.

Evans RG, Nesbit ME, Gehan EA, et al. Multimodality therapy for the management of localized Ewing's sarcoma of pelvic and sacral bones: a report from the second intergroup study. *Journal of Clinical Oncology.* 1991;9:1173–1180.

Faderl S, Kantarjian HM, and Talpaz M. Chronic myelogenous leukemia: update on biology and treatment. *Oncology.* 1999;13(2):169–184.

Fisher B, Dignam J, Wolmark N, et al. Tamoxifen and chemotherapy for lymph node–negative, estrogen receptor–positive breast cancer. *Journal of the National Cancer Institute.* 1997;89(22):1673–1682.

Giaccone G. New drugs for the management of lung cancer. *British Journal of Hospital Medicine.* 1996;55:634–638.

Glimelius B, Hoffman K, Graf W, et al. Quality of life during chemotherapy in patients with symptomatic advanced colorectal cancer. *Cancer.* 1994;73(3):556–562.

Greenblatt MS, Bennett WP, Hollstein M, and Harris CC. Mutations in the *p53* tumor suppressor gene: clues to cancer etiology and molecular pathogenesis. *Cancer Research.* 1994;54:4855.

Grier HE. The Ewing family of tumors: Ewing's sarcoma and primitive neuroectodermal tumors. *Pediatric Clinics of North America.* 1997;44(4):991–1004.

Grunberg SM and Hesketh PJ. Control of chemotherapy-induced nausea and vomiting. *New England Journal of Medicine.* 1993;329(24):1790–1796.

Guilhot F, Chastang C, Michallet M, et al. Interferon alpha-2b combined with cytarabine versus interferon alone in chronic myelogenous leukemia. *New England Journal of Medicine.* 1997;337(4):223–229.

Jackman AL, Boyle FT, and Harrap KR. Tomudex (ZD1694): From concept to care, a programme in rational drug discovery. *Investigational New Drugs.* 1996;14(3):305–316.

Jaffee EM and Greten TF. Cancer vaccines. *Journal of Clinical Oncology.* 1999;17(3):1047–1060.

Johnson DH, Turrisi AT, and Pass HI. Combined modality treatment for locally advanced non-small-cell lung cancer. In: Pass HI, Mitchell JB, Johnson DH, and Turrisi AT, eds. *Lung Cancer: Principles and Practice.* Philadelphia: Lippincott-Raven. 1996:863–874.

Kantarjian HM, Deisseroth A, Kurzrock R, et al. Chronic myelogenous leukemia: a concise update. *Blood.* 1993;82(3):691–703.

Kirsch DG and Kaston MD. Tumor-suppressor *p53*: implications for tumor development and prognosis. *Journal of Clinical Oncology.* 1998;16(9): 3158–3168.

Kressner U, Inganas M, Byding S, et al. Prognostic value of *p53* genetic changes in colorectal cancer. *Journal of Clinical Oncology.* 1999;17(2):593–599.

Levine AJ, Momand J, and Finlay CA. The *p53* tumor suppressor gene. *Nature.* 1991;351:453–456.

Lum LG. T cell–based immunotherapy for cancer: A virtual reality? *CA: A Cancer Journal for Clinicians.* 1999;49(2):74–100.

Kressner U, Inganäs M, Byding S, et al. Prognostic value of *p53* genetic changes in colorectal cancer. *Journal of Clinical Oncology.* 1999;17(2):593–599.

Macdonald JS. Adjuvant therapy for colon cancer. *CA: A Cancer Journal for Clinicians.* 1997;47(4):243–256.

Manning FCR and Patierno SR. Apoptosis: inhibitor or instigator of carcinogenesis? *Cancer Investigation.* 1996;14(5):455–465.

Mayer RJ and Schnipper LE. Correspondence. *New England Journal of Medicine.* 1997;337(13):935.

McCormick F. Cancer therapy based on p53. *The Cancer Journal.* 1999; 5(3):139–144.

McLaughlin P, Grillo-Lopez AJ, Link BK, et al. Rituximab chimeric anti-CD20 monoclonal antibody therapy for relapsed indolent lymphoma: half of patients respond to a four-dose treatment program. *Journal of Clinical Oncology.* 1998;16(8):2825–2833.

McLaughlin P, White CA, Grillo-Lopez AJ, and Maloney DG. Clinical status and optimal use of rituximab for B-cell lymphomas. *Oncology.* 1998; 12(12):1763–1769.

Slamon D, Leyland-Jones B, Wolter J, et al. Overall survival (OS) advantage to simultaneous chemotherapy (CRx) plus the humanized anti-HER2 monoclonal antibody Herceptin (H) in HER2-overexpressing (HER2+) metastatic breast cancer (MBC). *Proceedings of the American Society of Clinical Oncology.* 1999, #483.

Mendelsohn J. Principles of neoplasia. In: Isselbacher KJ, Braunwald E, Wilson JD, et al, eds. *Harrison's Principles of Internal Medicine.* [13th edition] New York: McGraw-Hill. 1994:1814–1826.

Olivotto IA, Badjik CD, Plenderleith IH, et al. Adjuvant systemic therapy and survival after breast cancer. *New England Journal of Medicine.* 1994;330(12):805–810.

Overgaard M, Hansen PS, Overgaard J, et al. Postoperative radiotherapy in high-risk premenopausal women with breast cancer who receive adjuvant chemotherapy. *New England Journal of Medicine.* 1997;337(14):949–955.

Pegram MD, Lipton A, Hayes DF, et al. Phase II study of receptor-enhanced chemosensitivity using recombinant humanized anti-p185[HER2/neu] monoclonal antibody plus cisplatin in patients with HER2/*neu*-overexpressing metastatic breast cancer refractory to chemotherapy treatment. *Journal of Clinical Oncology.* 1998;16(8):2659–2671.

Peters KF and Hadley DW. The Human Genome Project. *Cancer Nursing.* 1997;20(1):62–71.

Portenoy RK and Lesage P. Trends in cancer pain management. *Cancer Control.* 1999;6(2):136–145.

Punt CJA. New drugs in the treatment of colorectal carcinoma. *Cancer.* 1998; 83(4):679–689.

Ragaz J, Jackson SM, Le N, et al. Adjuvant radiotherapy and chemotherapy in node-positive premenopausal women with breast cancer. *New England Journal of Medicine.* 1997;337(14):956–962.

Reed JC. Dysregulation of apoptosis in cancer. *Journal of Clinical Oncology.* 1999;17(9):2941–2953.

Rosen G, Forscher CA, Mankin HJ, and Selch MT. Bone tumors. In: Holland JF, Frei E, Bast RC, et al, eds. *Cancer Medicine.* [4th edition] Baltimore: Williams and Wilkins. 1997:2503–2557.

Ruckdeschel JC and Robinson LA. Non-small-cell lung cancer: surgery and post-operative adjuvant chemotherapy. In: Pass HI, Mitchell JB, Johnson DH, and Turrisi AT, eds. *Lung Cancer: Principles and Practice.* Philadelphia: Lippincott-Raven. 1996:839–850.

Schiffer CA. Acute myeloid leukemia in adults. In: Holland JF, Frei E, Bast RC, et al, eds. *Cancer Medicine.* [4th edition] Baltimore: Williams and Wilkins. 1997:2617–2649.

Seshadri R, Firgaira FA, Horsfall DJ, et al. Clinical significance of HER-2/*neu* oncogene amplification in primary breast cancer. *Journal of Clinical Oncology.* 1993;11:1936–1942.

Shepherd FA. Chemotherapy for non-small-cell lung cancer: Have we reached a new plateau? *Seminars in Oncology.* 1999;26(1)supplement4:3–11.

Slamon DJ, Clark GM, Wong SG, et al. Human breast cancer: Correlation of relapse and survival with amplification of the HER-2/*neu* oncogene. *Science.* 1987;235:177–182.

Slamon DJ, Godolphin W, Jones LA, et al. Studies of the HER-2/*neu* proto-oncogene in human breast and ovarian cancer. *Science.* 1989;244:707–712.

Stat Bite: Persons living with major cancers in the United States, 1998. *Journal of the National Cancer Institute.* 1998;90(8):565.

Stewart BW. Mechanisms of apoptosis: integration of genetic, biochemical, and cellular indicators. *Journal of the National Cancer Institute.* 1994;86(17): 1286–1296.

Suit H, Isselbacher K, and Chabner B. Correspondence. *New England Journal of Medicine.* 1997;337(13):936–937.

Talpaz M, Kantarjian H, Kurzrock R, et al. Interferon-alpha produces sustained cytogenetic responses in chronic myelogenous leukemia. *Annals of Internal Medicine.* 1991;114(7):532–538.

Van Houtte PJ. Non-small-cell lung cancer: surgery and postoperative radiation. In: Pass HI, Mitchell JB, Johnson DH, and Turrisi AT, eds. *Lung Cancer: Principles and Practice.* Philadelphia: Lippincott-Raven. 1996:851–862.

Velders MP, Schreiber H, and Kast WM. Active immunization against cancer cells: impediments and advances. *Seminars in Oncology.* 1998;25(6):697–706.

Vesole DH, Jagannath S, Tricot G, et al. Autologous bone marrow and peripheral blood stem cell transplantation in multiple myeloma. *Cancer Investigation.* 1996;14(4):378–391.

Vose J and Armitage JO. Clinical applications of hematopoietic growth factors. *Journal of Clinical Oncology.* 1995;13(4):1023–1035.

Wolmark N, Rockette H, Fisher B, et al. The benefit of leucovorin-modulated fluorouracil as postoperative adjuvant therapy for primary colon cancer: results from the national surgical adjuvant breast and bowel project protocol C-03. *New England Journal of Medicine.* 1993;11(10):1879–1887.

CHAPTER 4: EDUCATION AND INFORMATION

A Century of Oncology. A photographic history of cancer research and therapy. With commentary by J. Lynne Dodson. Greenwich, CT: Greenwich Press. 1997.

Abeloff MD, Armitage JO, Lichter AS, and Niederhuber JE, eds. *Clinical Oncology.* New York: Churchill Livingstone. 1995.

Albertsen PC. Prostate disease in older men: 2. Cancer. *Hospital Practice.* October 15, 1997: 159–181.

American College of Physicians. Screening for Prostate Cancer. *Annals of Internal Medicine.* 1997;126(6):480–484.

Balmer JA. Alternative cancer therapy resources on the Internet. *Highlights in Oncology Practice.* 1998;15(4):110–113.

Bates SE. Clinical application of serum tumor markers. *Annals of Internal Medicine.* 1990;115(8):623–638.

Bick RL, guest ed. Paraneoplastic syndromes. *Hematology/Oncology Clinics of North America.* 1996;10(4).

Biermann JS, Golladay GJ, Greenfield ML, and Baker LH. Evaluation of cancer information on the Internet. *Cancer*. 1999;86(3):381–390.

Bonadonna G, Valagussa P, Moliterni A, et al. Adjuvant cyclophosphamide, methotrexate, and fluorouracil in node-positive breast cancer: the results of 20 years of follow-up. *New England Journal of Medicine*. 1995;332(14):901–906.

Brinton LA and Hoover RN. Epidemiology of gynecologic cancers. In: *Principles and Practice of Gynecologic Oncology*. Hoskins WJ, Perez CA, and Young R, eds. [2nd edition] Philadelphia: Lippincott-Raven. 1997:3–29.

Burnet FM. Immunological surveillance in neoplasia. *Transplantation Review*. 1971;7:3–25.

Cannistra SA. Cancer of the ovary. *New England Journal of Medicine*. 1993; 329(21):1550–1559.

Carney DN. New agents in the management of advanced non-small-cell lung cancer. *Seminars in Oncology*. 1998;25(4)supplement9:83–88.

Catalona WJ, Partin AW, Slawin KM, et al. Use of the percentage of free prostate-specific antigen to enhance differentiation of prostate cancer from benign prostatic disease. *Journal of the American Medical Association*. 1998;279(19):1542–1547.

Closing in on Cancer: Solving a 5000-Year-Old Mystery. A publication of The National Cancer Institute. U.S. Department of Health and Human Services. NIH Publication No. 98–2955. 1998.

Colditz GA, Hankinson SE, Hunter DJ, et al. The use of estrogens and progestins and the risk of breast cancer in postmenopausal women. *New England Journal of Medicine*. 1995;332(24):1589–1593.

Colditz GA, Willett WC, Hunter DJ, et al. Family history, age, and risk of breast cancer. *Journal of the American Medical Association*. 1993;270(3):338–343.

Cody HS. Sentinel lymph node mapping in breast cancer. *Oncology*. 1999; 13(1):25–34.

D'Amico AV, Whittington R, Malkowitz B, et al. Biochemical outcome after radical prostatectomy, external beam radiation therapy, or interstitial radiation therapy for clinically localized prostate cancer. *Journal of the American Medical Association*. 1998;280(11):969–974.

DeVita VT, Hellman S, and Rosenberg SA., eds. *Cancer: Principles and practice of oncology*. [5th edition] Philadelphia: Lippincott-Raven. 1997.

Pergament D, Pergament E, Wonderlick A, and Fiddler M. At the crossroads: the intersection of the Internet and clinical oncology. *Oncology*. 1999;13(4):577–583.

Fisher B, Bauer M, Margolese R, et al. Five-year results of a randomized clinical trial comparing total mastectomy and segmental mastectomy with or without radiation in the treatment of breast cancer. *New England Journal of Medicine*. 1985;312:665–673.

Fisher B, Dignam J, Wolmark N, et al. Tamoxifen and chemotherapy for lymph node–negative, estrogen receptor–positive breast cancer. *Journal of the National Cancer Institute*. 1997;89(22):1673–1682.

Garcia-Martinez C, Costelli P, Lopez-Soriano FJ, and Argiles JM. Is TNF really involved in cachexia? *Cancer Investigation*. 1997;15(1):47–54.

Giles G, Ireland P. Diet, nutrition and prostate cancer. *International Journal of Cancer*. 1997;suppl 10:13–17.

Glode LM. Challenges and opportunities of the Internet for medical oncology. *Journal of Clinical Oncology*. 1996;14(7):2181–2186.

Greene MH. Genetics of breast cancer. *Mayo Clinic Proceedings*. 1997;72: 54–65.

Grove A. Taking on prostate cancer. *Fortune*. May 13, 1996. Page 55.

Guiliano AE, Jones RC, Brennan M, and Statman R. Sentinel lymphadenectomy in breast cancer. *Journal of Clinical Oncology*. 1997;15(6):2345–2350.

Hamilton AB. Psychological aspects of ovarian cancer. *Cancer Investigation*. 1999;17(5):335–341.

Harris KA. The informational needs of patients with cancer and their families. *Cancer Practice*. 1998;6(1):39–46.

Henderson IC. Risk factors for breast cancer development. *Cancer*. (Supplement) 1993;71(6): 2127–2140.

Henschke CI, McCauley DI, Yankelevitz DF, et al. Early lung cancer action project: overall design and findings from baseline screening. *The Lancet*. 1999;354:888–891.

Hewitt HB, Blake ER, and Walder AS. A critique of the evidence for active host defense against cancer, based on studies of 27 murine tumors of spontaneous origin. *British Journal of Cancer*. 1976;33:241–259.

Holland JF, Frei E, Bast RC, et al, eds. *Cancer Medicine*. [4th edition] Baltimore: Williams and Wilkins. 1997.

Huang Z, Hankinson SE, Colditz GA, et al. Dual effects of weight and weight gain on breast cancer risk. *Journal of the American Medical Association*. 1997;278(17):1407–1411.

Hunter DJ, Spiegelman D, Adami HO, et al. Cohort studies of fat intake and the risk of breast cancer—a pooled analysis. *New England Journal of Medicine*. 1996;334(6):356–361.

Jacobs I and Bast RC. The CA-125 tumor-associated antigen: A review of the literature. *Human Reproduction*. 1989;4:1–12.

Jacobsen SJ, Katusic SK, Bergstralh MS, et al. Incidence of prostate cancer diagnosis in the eras before and after serum prostate-specific antigen testing. *Journal of the American Medical Association*. 1995;274(18):1445–1449.

Kempin SJ. Hemostatic defects in cancer patients. *Cancer Investigation*. 1997; 15(1):23–36.

King SE and Schottenfeld D. The "epidemic" of breast cancer in the U.S.—determining the factors. *Oncology.* 1996;10(4):453–462.

Kolonel LN, Nomura AM, and Cooney RV. Dietary fat and prostate cancer: current status. *Journal of the National Cancer Institute.* 1999;91(5):414–428.

Landis SH, Murray T, Bolden S, and Wingo PA. Cancer Statistics, 1999. *CA: A Cancer Journal for Clinicians.* 1999;49(1):8–31.

McGuire WP, Hoskins WJ, Brady MF, et al. Cyclophosphamide and cisplatin compared with paclitaxel and cisplatin in patients with stage III and stage IV ovarian cancer. *New England Journal of Medicine.* 1996;334(1):1–6

Mott K. Cancer and the Internet. *Newsweek.* August 19, 1996. Page 19.

Murphy GP, Barren RJ, Erickson SJ, et al. Evaluation and comparison of two new prostate carcinoma markers. *Cancer.* 1996;78(4):809–818.

Nachman RL and Silverstein R. Hypercoagulable states. *Annals of Internal Medicine.* 1993;119(8):819–827.

Nelson KA, Walsh D, and Sheehan FA. The cancer-anorexia syndrome. *Journal of Clinical Oncology.* 1994;12(1):213–225.

Olivotto IA, Badjik CD, Plenderleith IH, et al. Adjuvant systemic therapy and survival after breast cancer. *New England Journal of Medicine.* 1994;330(12):805–810.

O'Rourke ME. Narrowing the options: the process of deciding on prostate cancer treatment. *Cancer Investigation.* 1999;17(5):349–359.

Ottery FD, Walsh D, and Strawford A. Pharmacologic management of anorexia/cachexia. *Seminars in Oncology.* 1998;25(2)supplement6:35–44.

Ozols RF. Treatment of ovarian cancer: current status. *Seminars in Oncology.* 1994;21(2)supplement2:1–10.

Ozols RF, Rubin AC, Thomas G, and Robboy S. Epithelial ovarian cancer. In: *Principles and Practice of Gynecologic Oncology.* Hoskins WJ, Perez CA, and Young R, eds. [2nd edition] Philadelphia: Lippincott-Raven. 1997:919–986.

Pass HI, Mitchell JB, Johnson DH, and Turrisi AT, eds. *Lung Cancer: Principles and Practice.* Philadelphia: Lippincott-Raven. 1996.

Rao AK, Rubin RN. Hypercoagulable states. *Hem/Onc Annals.* 1993;1(2):138–146.

Raven RW. *The Theory and Practice of Oncology. Historical evolution and present principles.* New Jersey: The Parthenon Publishing Group, Inc. 1990.

Rosenthal A and Jacobs I. Ovarian cancer screening. *Seminars in Oncology.* 1998;25(3):315–325.

Schuurman AG, van den Brandt PA, Dorant E., et al. Association of energy and fat intake with prostate carcinoma risk. *Cancer.* 1999;86(6):1019–1027.

Smith-Warner SA, Spiegelman D, Yuan SS, et al. Alcohol and breast cancer in women. A pooled analysis of cohort studies. *Journal of the American Medical Association.* 1998;279(7):535–540.

Sikorski R and Peters R. Oncology ASAP: where to find reliable information on the Internet. *Journal of the American Medical Association.* 1997;277(18): 1431–1432.

Solin LJ, Fox K, August DA, et al. Breast cancer. In: *Principles and Practice of Gynecologic Oncology.* Hoskins WJ, Perez CA, and Young R, eds. [2nd edition] Philadelphia: Lippincott-Raven. 1997:1079–1142.

Stanford JL, Weiss NS, Voigt LF, et al. Combined estrogen and progestin hormone replacement therapy in relation to risk of breast cancer in middle-aged women. *Journal of the American Medical Association.* 1995;274(2):137–142.

Stutman O. Cancer. In: Nelsen DS, ed. *Natural Immunity.* Sydney, Australia: Academic Press. 1989:479–494.

Veronesi U, Luini A, Del Vecchio M, et al. Radiotherapy after breast-preserving surgery in women with localized cancer of the breast. *New England Journal of Medicine.* 1993;328(22):1587–1591.

von Eschenbach A, Ho R, Murphy G, et al. American Cancer Society guideline for the early detection of prostate cancer: Update 1997. *CA: A Cancer Journal for Clinicians.* 1997;47(5):261–264.

Warmuth MA, Sutton LM, and Winer EP. A review of hereditary breast cancer: From screening to risk factor modification. *American Journal of Medicine.* 1997;102:407–415.

Wood MS and Delozier EP. *Cancer resources on the Internet.* Binghamton, NY: The Haworth Press. 1997.

Wu AH, Pike MC, and Stram DO. Meta-analysis: dietary fat intake, serum estrogen levels, and the risk of breast cancer. *Journal of the National Cancer Institute.* 1999;91(6)529–534.

Yip I, Heber D, and Aronson W. Nutrition and prostate cancer. *Urologic Clinics of North America.* 1999;26(2):403–411.

Zhang S, Hunter DJ, Forman MR, et al. Dietary carotenoids and vitamins A, C, and E and risk of breast cancer. *Journal of the National Cancer Institute.* 1999;91(6):547–556.

CHAPTER 5: PSYCHOSOCIAL SUPPORT

Berkmann LF and Syme SL. Social networks, host resistance, and mortality. *American Journal of Epidemiology.* 1979;109:186–204.

Cassileth BR, Lusk EJ, Miller DS, et al. Psychosocial correlates of survival in advanced malignant disease? *New England Journal of Medicine.* 1985; 312(24):1551–1555.

Cohen S, Doyle WJ, Skoner DP, et al. Social ties and susceptibility to the common cold. *Journal of the American Medical Association.* 1997;277(24): 1940–1944.

Coluzzi PH, Grant M, Doroshow JH, et al. Survey of the provision of supportive care services at National Cancer Institute–designated cancer centers. *Journal of Clinical Oncology.* 1995;13(3):756–764.

Coreil J and Behal R. Man to man prostate cancer support groups. *Cancer Practice.* 1999;7(3):122–129.

Creagan ET. Attitude and disposition: Do they make a difference in cancer survival? *Mayo Clinic Proceedings.* 1997;72:160–164.

Dreher H. The scientific and moral imperative for broad-based psychosocial interventions for cancer. *Advances: The Journal of Mind-Body Health.* 1997; 13(3):38–49.

Fawzy FI, Cousins N, Fawzy NW, et al. A structured psychiatric intervention for cancer patients. I. Changes over time in methods of coping and affective disturbance. *Archives of General Psychiatry.* 1990;47:720–725.

Fawzy FI, Fawzy NW, Arndt LA, et al. Critical review of pyschosocial interventions in cancer care. *Archives in General Psychiatry.* 1995;52:100–113.

Fawzy FI, Fawzy NW, Hyun CS, et al. Malignant melanoma: Effects of an early structured psychiatric intervention, coping, and affective state on recurrence and survival 6 years later. *Archives of General Psychiatry.* 1993;50:681–689.

Fawzy FI, Kemeny ME, Fawzy NW, et al. A structured psychiatric intervention for cancer patients. II. Changes over time in immunologic measures. *Archives of General Psychiatry.* 1990;47:729–735.

Fobair P. Cancer support groups and group therapies: Part I. Historical and theoretical background and research on effectiveness. *Journal of Psychosocial Oncology.* 1997;15(1):63–81.

Fox BH. The role of psychological factors in cancer incidence and prognosis. *Cancer.* 1995;9(3):245–253.

Gellert GA, Maxwell RM, and Siegel BS. Survival of breast cancer patients receiving adjunctive psychosocial support therapy: A 10-year follow-up study. *Journal of Clinical Oncology.* 1993;11(1):66–69.

Goodwin JS, Hunt WC, Key CR, and Samet JM. The effect of marital status on stage, treatment, and survival of cancer patients. *Journal of the American Medical Association.* 1987;258(21):3125–3130.

Holland JC and Breitbart W, eds. *Psychooncology.* New York: Oxford University Press. 1998.

Holland JC and Rowland JH, eds. *Handbook of Psychooncology: Psychological Care of the Patient with Cancer.* New York: Oxford University Press. 1990.

Horowitz S. The power of more than one: the role of support groups in mind-body healing. *Alternative and Complementary Therapies.* 1998;4(2):84–88.

House JS, Landis KR, and Umberson D. Social relationships and health. *Science.* 1988;241:540–545.

Kogon MM, Biswas A, Pearl D, et al. Effects of medical and psychotherapeutic treatment on the survival of women with metastatic breast carcinoma. *Cancer.* 1997;80(2):225–230.

Krizek C, Roberts, C, Ragan R, et al. Gender and cancer support group participation. *Cancer Practice.* 1999;7(2):86–92.

Leedham B and Ganz PA. Psychosocial concerns and quality of life in breast cancer survivors. *Cancer Investigation.* 1999;17(5):342–348.

Manne S. Cancer in the marital context: a review of the literature. *Cancer Investigation.* 1998;16(3):188–202.

Maunsell E, Brisson J, and Deschenes L. Social support and survival among women with breast cancer. *Cancer.* 1995;76(4):631–637.

Meyerowitz BE, Heinrich R, and Coscarelli Schag CA. Helping patients cope with cancer. *Oncology.* 1989;3(11):120–131.

Richardson JL, Shelton DR, Krailo M, and Levine AM. The effect of compliance with treatment on survival among patients with hematologic malignancies. *Journal of Clinical Oncology.* 1990;8(2):356–364.

Shrock D, Palmer RF, and Taylor B. Effects of psychosocial intervention on survival among patients with stage I breast and prostate cancer: a matched case-controlled study. *Alternative Therapies in Health and Medicine.* 1999;5(3):49–55.

Simonton SS and Sherman AC. Psychological aspects of mind-body medicine: promises and pitfalls from research with cancer patients. *Alternative Therapies in Health and Medicine.* 1998;4(4):50–67.

Spiegel D. *Living Beyond Limits: New Hope and Help for Facing Life-Threatening Illness.* New York: Times Books. 1993.

Spiegel D. Psychosocial interventions in cancer. *Journal of the National Cancer Institute.* 1993;85(15):1198–1205.

Spiegel D. Health caring: psychosocial support for patients with cancer. *Cancer.* 1994;74(4)supplement:1453–1457.

Spiegel D. Psychological distress and disease course for women with breast cancer: one answer, many questions. [editorial] *Journal of the National Cancer Institute.* 1996;88(10):629–631.

Spiegel D, Bloom JR, Kraemer HC, and Gottheil E. Effect of psychosocial treatment on survival of patients with metastatic cancer. *The Lancet.* 1989; 2:888–891.

Spiegel D, Morrow GR, Classen C, et al. Effects of group therapy on women with primary breast cancer. *The Breast Journal.* 1996;2(1):104–106.

Tross S, Herndon J, Korzun A, et al. Psychological symptoms and disease-free and overall survival in women with stage II breast cancer. *Journal of the National Cancer Institute.* 1996;88(10):661–667.

CHAPTER 6: THE BODY AS GARDEN

Alberts DS and Garcia DJ. An overview of clinical cancer chemoprevention studies, with emphasis on positive phase III studies. *Journal of Nutrition.* 1995; 125:692s–697s.

ASCO Special Article. The physician and unorthodox cancer therapies. *Journal of Clinical Oncology.* 1997;15(1):401–406.

Alphen JV and Aris A, eds. *Oriental Medicine: An Illustrated Guide to the Asian Arts of Healing.* Boston: Shambhala. 1996.

Barrett S and Herbert VD. Questionable cancer therapies. In: Holland JF, Frei E, Bast RC, et al, eds. *Cancer Medicine.* [4th edition] Baltimore: Williams and Wilkins. 1997:1459–1467.

Beinfeld H and Corngold E. *Between Heaven and Earth: A Guide to Chinese Medicine.* New York, NY: Ballantine. 1992.

Boik J. *Cancer and Natural Medicine: A Textbook of Basic Science and Clinical Research.* Princeton, MN: Oregon Medical Press. 1996.

Bland KI. Quality-of-life management for cancer patients. *CA—A Journal for Clinicians.* 1997; 47(4):194–238.

Buckner JC, Malkin MG, Reed E, et al. Phase II study of antineoplastons A10 (NSC 648539) and AS2–1 (NSC 620261) in patients with recurrent glioma. *Mayo Clinic Proceedings.* 1999;74:137–145.

Bushman JL. Green tea and cancer in humans: a review of the literature. *Nutrition and Cancer.* 1998;31(3):151–159.

Burstein HJ, Gelber S, Gaudagnoli E, and Weeks JC. Use of alternative medicine by women with early-stage breast cancer. *New England Journal of Medicine.* 1999;340(22):1733–1739.

Cassileth BR. *The Alternative Medicine Handbook: The Complete Reference Guide to Alternative and Complementary Therapies.* New York: W.W. Norton and Company. 1998.

Cassileth BR. What every oncologist should know about alternative medicine. *Contemporary Oncology.* February 1994:24–38.

Cassileth BR. Unorthodox cancer medicine. *Cancer Investigation.* 1986;4(6): 591–598.

Cassileth BR and Chapman CC. Alternative and complementary cancer therapies. *Cancer.* 1996;77(6):1026–1034.

Cassileth BR, Lusk EJ, Guerry D, et al. Survival and quality of life among patients receiving unproven as compared with conventional cancer therapy. *New England Journal of Medicine.* 1991;324(17)1180–1185.

Cassileth BR, Lusk EJ, Strouse TB, and Bodebheimer BJ. Contemporary unorthodox treatments in cancer medicine: a study of patients, treatments and practitioners. *Annals of Internal Medicine.* 1984;101(1):105–112.

Cella DF and Tulsky DS. Quality of life in cancer: definition, purpose, and method of measurement. *Cancer Investigation*. 1993;11(3):327–336.

Chiu BCH, Cerhan JR, Folsom AR, et al. Diet and risk of non-Hodgkin lymphoma in older women. *Journal of the American Medical Association*. 1996;275(17):1315–1321.

Clark LC, Combs GF, Turnbull BW, et al. Effects of selenium supplementation for cancer prevention in patients with carcinoma of the skin: a randomized controlled trial. *Journal of the American Medical Association*. 1996;276(24): 1957–1963.

Clifford, Terry. *Tibetan Buddhist Medicine and Psychiatry: The Diamond Healing*. York Beach, ME: Samuel Weiser, Inc. 1984.

Coker KH. Meditation and prostate cancer: Integrating a mind/body intervention with traditional therapies. *Seminars in Urologic Oncology*. 1999;17(2): 111–118.

Clinton SK and Giovannucci EL. Nutrition in the etiology and prevention of cancer. In: Holland JF, Frei E, Bast RC, et al, eds. *Cancer Medicine*. [4th edition] Baltimore: Williams and Wilkins. 1997:465–494.

Cohen SR, Mount BM, Tomas JJN, and Mount LF. Existential well-being is an important determinant of quality of life. *Cancer*. 1996;77(3):576–586.

Colditz GA. Selenium and cancer prevention: Promising results indicate further trials required. *Journal of the American Medical Association*. 1996;276(24):1984–1985.

Clinton SK and Giovannucci EL. Nutrition in the etiology and prevention of cancer. In: Holland JF, Frei E, Bast RC, et al, eds. *Cancer Medicine*. [4th edition] Baltimore: Williams and Wilkins. 1997:465–494.

Courneya KS and Friedenreich CM. Relationship between exercise pattern across the cancer experience and current quality of life in colorectal cancer survivors. *Journal of Alternative and Complementary Medicine*. 1997;3(3): 215–226.

Dimeo FC, Tilmann MHM, Bertz H, et al. Aerobic exercise in the rehabilitation of cancer patients after high dose chemotherapy and autologous peripheral stem cell transplantation. *Cancer*. 1997;79(9):1717–1722.

DiPaola RS, Zhang H, Lambert GH, et al. Clinical and biological activity of an estrogenic herbal combination (PC-SPES) in prostate cancer. *New England Journal of Medicine*. 1998;339(12):785.

Donden Y. *Health Through Balance: An Introduction to Tibetan Medicine*. Ithaca, NY: Snow Lion Publications. 1986.

Dorgan JF, Stanczyk FZ, Longcope C, et al. Relationship of serum dehydroepiandrosterone (DHEA), DHEA-sulfate, and 5-androstene-3 beta, 17 beta-diol to risk of breast cancer in postmenopausal women. *Cancer Epidemiology, Biomarkers, and Prevention*. 1997;6(3):177–181.

Downer SM, Cody MM, McCluskay P, et al. Pursuit and practice of complementary therapies by cancer patients receiving conventional treatment. *British Medical Journal.* 1994;309:86–89.

Eaton NE, Reeves GK, Appleby PN, and Key TJ. Endogenous sex hormones and prostate cancer: a quantitative review of prospective studies. *British Journal of Cancer.* 1999;80(7):930–934.

Fenton P. In the realm of the Medicine Buddha. *Shambhala Sun.* January 1998:50–57.

Ferrell BR, Grant M, Funk B, et al. Quality of life in breast cancer. *Cancer Practice.* 1996;4(6):331–340.

Field T, Ironson G, Scafidi F, et al. Massage therapy is associated with enhancement of the immune system's cytotoxic capacity. *International Journal of Neuroscience.* 1996;84(1–4):205–217.

Field T, Ironson G, Scafidi F, et al. Massage therapy reduces anxiety and enhances EEG pattern of alertness and math computations. *International Journal of Neuroscience.* 1996;86(3–4):197–205.

Finckh E. *Foundations of Tibetan Medicine, According to the Book rGyud bzi. Volume One.* London: Robinson and Watkins Books, Ltd. 1978.

Finckh E. *Foundations of Tibetan Medicine, According to the Book rGyud bzi. Volume Two.* Longmead, England: Element Books, Ltd. 1988.

Franceschi S, Favero A, Decarli A, et al. Intake of micronutrients and risk of breast cancer. *The Lancet.* 1996;347:1351–1356.

Frawley D. *Ayurvedic Healing: A Comprehensive Guide.* Salt Lake City: Passage Press. 1989.

Fuchs CS, Giovannucci EL, Colditz GA, et al. Dietary fiber and the risk of colorectal cancer and adenoma in women. *New England Journal of Medicine.* 1999;340(3):169–176.

Ganz PA. Quality of life and the patient with cancer: Individual and policy implications. *Cancer.* 1994;74(4)supplement:1445–1452.

Giles G, Ireland P. Diet, nutrition and prostate cancer. *International Journal of Cancer.* 1997;supplement 10:13–17.

Geffen JR. Traditional medicine in the Himalayas of Nepal. *New York University Physician.* 1985;41(2):58–67.

Greenberg ER and Sporn MB. Antioxidant vitamins, cancer, and cardiovascular disease. [editorial] *The New England Journal of Medicine.* 1996;334(18):1189–1190.

Greenwald P and McDonald SS. Cancer prevention: The roles of diet and chemoprevention. *Cancer Control.* 1997;4(2):118–127.

Grindel CG, Whitmer K, and Barsevik A. Quality of life and nutritional support in patients with cancer. *Cancer Practice.* 1996;4(2):81–87.

Hartwell JL. *Plants Used Against Cancer*. Lawrence, MA: Quarterman Publications, Inc. 1982.

Hauser SP. Unproven methods in cancer treatment. *Current Opinion in Oncology*. 1993;5:646–654.

Hennekens CH, Buring JE, Manson JE, et al. Lack of effect of long-term supplementation with beta carotene on the incidence of malignant neoplasms and cardiovascular disease. *New England Journal of Medicine*. 1996;334(18): 1145–1149.

Hensrud DD, Engle DD, and Scheitel SM. Underreporting the use of dietary supplements and non-prescription medications among patients undergoing a periodic health examination. *Mayo Clinic Proceedings*. 1999;74:443–447.

Herbert V. Unproven (questionable) dietary and nutritional methods in cancer prevention and treatment. *Cancer*. 1986;58:1930–1941.

Hiltebrand EU and Annala S. Adjunctive psychosocial support as a complement to traditional medical interventions for the cancer population. *Cancer Management*. 1998;3(1):20–28.

Holmes MD, Hunter DJ, Colditz GA, et al. Association of dietary intake of fat and fatty acids with risk of breast cancer. *Journal of the American Medical Association*. 1999;281(10):914–920.

Holmes MD, Stampfer MJ, Colditz GA, et al. Dietary factors and the survival of women with breast carcinoma. *Cancer*. 1999;86(5):826–835.

Holt S. Chemoprevention of cancer with green tea. *Alternative and Complementary Therapies*. 1998;4(1):48–52.

Hunter DJ, Spiegelman D, Adami HO, et al. Cohort studies of fat intake and the risk of breast cancer—a pooled analysis. *New England Journal of Medicine*. 1996;334(6):356–361.

Jones JA, Nguyen A, Straub M, et al. Use of DHEA in a patient with advanced prostate cancer: a case report and review. *Urology*. 1997;50(5):784–788.

Kaptchuk TJ. *The Web That Has No Weaver: Understanding Chinese Medicine*. New York: Congdon and Weed. 1983.

Kosty MP, Fleishman SB, Herndon JE, et al. Cisplatin, vinblastine, and hydrazine sulfate in advanced, non-small-cell lung cancer: a randomized placebo-controlled, double-blind phase III study of the Cancer and Leukemia Group B. *Journal of Clinical Oncology*. 1994;12(6):1113–1120.

Krieg MB. *Green Medicine: The Search for Plants That Heal*. Chicago: Rand McNally & Company. 1964.

Labrie F, Bélanger A, Van LT, et al. DHEA and the intracrine formation of androgens and estrogens in peripheral target tissues: its role during aging. *Steroids*. 1998;63(5–6):322–328.

Labriola D and Livingston R. Possible interactions between dietary antioxidants and chemotherapy. *Oncology.* 1999;13(7):1003–1008.

Lad V. An introduction to Ayurveda. *Alternative Therapies in Health and Medicine.* 1995;1(3):57–63.

Lad V. *Ayurveda: The Science of Self-Healing.* Santa Fe, NM: Lotus Press. 1984.

Lerner M. *Choices in Healing: Integrating the Best of Conventional and Complementary Approaches to Cancer.* Cambridge, MA: The MIT Press. 1994.

Loizzo JJ and Blackhall LJ. Traditional alternatives as complementary sciences: the case of Indo-Tibetan medicine. *Journal of Alternative and Complementary Medicine.* 1998;4(3):311–319.

Loprinzi CL, Goldberg RM, Su JQ, et al. Placebo-controlled trial of hydrazine sulfate in patients with newly diagnosed non-small-cell lung cancer. *Journal of Clinical Oncology.* 1994;12(6):1126–1129.

Loprinzi CL, Kuross SA, O'Fallon JR, et al. Randomized placebo-controlled evaluation of hydrazine sulfate in patients with advanced colorectal cancer. *Journal of Clinical Oncology.* 1994;12(6):1121–1125.

McTiernan A, Ulrich C, Kumai C, et al. Anthropometric and hormone effects of an eight-week exercise-diet intervention in breast cancer patients: results of a pilot study. *Cancer Epidemiology, Biomarkers, and Prevention.* 1998;7(6):477–481.

Mendoza TR, Wang XS, Cleeland CS, et al. The rapid assessment of fatigue severity in cancer patients. *Cancer.* 1999;85(5):1186–1196.

Miller DR, Anderson GT, Stark JJ, et al. Phase I/II trial of the safety and efficacy of shark cartilage in the treatment of advanced cancer. *Journal of Clinical Oncology.* 1998;16(11):3649–3655.

Moertel CG, Fleming TR, Rubin J, et al. A clinical trial of amygdalin (Laetrile) in the treatment of human cancer. *New England Journal of Medicine.* 1982;306:201–206.

Moertel CG, Ames MM, Kovach JS, et al. A pharmacologic and toxicological study of amygdalin. *Journal of the American Medical Association.* 1981; 245:591–594.

Moss RW. *Herbs Against Cancer: History and Controversy.* Brooklyn, NY: Equinox Press, Inc. 1998.

Muir M. (Green) tea time: does it help prevent cancer? *Alternative and Complementary Therapies.* 1998;4(1):43–47.

Muir M. Alternative therapies for cancer-related fatigue. *Alternative and Complementary Therapies.* 1997;3(4):243–254.

Nelson WK. Alternative cancer treatments. *Highlights in Oncology Practice.* 1998;15(4):85–93.

Omenn GS, Goodman GE, Thornquist MD, et al. Effects of a combination of beta carotene and vitamin A on lung cancer and cardiovascular disease. *New England Journal of Medicine.* 1996;334(18):1150–1155.

Osoba D, Murray N, Gelman K, et al. Quality of life, appetite, and weight change in patients receiving dose-intensive chemotherapy. *Oncology.* 1994;8(4): 61–69.

Parfitt A. Acupuncture as an antiemetic treatment. *Journal of Alternative and Complementary Medicine.* 1996;2(1):167–173.

Patel V. Ayurveda: science of integrative approaches to health and disease. *Internal Journal of Integrative Medicine.* 1999;1(5):7–9.

Paulsen SM. Use of herbal products and dietary supplements by oncology patients— informed decisions? *Highlights in Oncology Practice.* 1998;15(4):94–106.

Pennebaker JW, Kiecolt-Glaser JK, and Glaser R. Disclosures of traumas and immune function: Health implications for psychotherapy. *Journal of Consulting and Clinical Psychology.* 1988;56:239–245.

Petire KJ, Booth RJ, et al. Disclosure of trauma and immune response to a hepatitis B vaccination program. *Journal of Consulting and Clinical Psychology.* 1995;63:787–792.

Pinto BM, Maruyama NC, Engebretson TO, and Thebarge RW. Participation in exercise, mood, and coping in survivors of early stage breast cancer. *Journal of Psychosocial Oncology.* 1998;16(2):45–58.

Quillan P. The ideal anti-cancer diet. *American Journal of Natural Medicine.* 1998;5(7):21–25.

Rinpoche S. The spiritual heart of Tibetan Medicine: Its contribution to the modern world. *Alternative Therapies in Health and Medicine.* 1999;5(3):70–72.

Segar ML, Katch VL, Roth RS, et al. The effects of aerobic exercise on self-esteem and depressive and anxiety symptoms among breast cancer survivors. *Oncology Nursing Forum.* 1998;25(1):107–113.

Serenson I. Integrated Chinese/Western therapies in the treatment of cancer, Part 1. *Alternative and Complementary Therapies.* 1997;3(6):441–446.

Serenson I. Integrated Chinese/Western therapies in the treatment of cancer, Part 2. *Alternative and Complementary Therapies.* 1998;4(2):134–138.

Shklar G. Mechanisms of cancer inhibition by anti-oxidant nutrients. *Oral Oncology.* 1998;34(1):24–29.

Singh DK and Lippman SM. Cancer chemoprevention—Part 1: Retinoids and carotenoids and other classic antioxidants. *Oncology.* 1998;12(11):1643–1658.

Singh DK and Lippman SM. Cancer chemoprevention—Part 2: Hormones, non-classic antioxidants, NSAID's, and other agents. *Oncology.* 1998;12(12):1787–1800.

Smith MC, Stallings MA, Mariner S, and Burrall M. Benefits of massage therapy in hospitalized patients: a descriptive and qualitative evaluation. *Alternative Therapies in Health and Medicine.* 1999;5(4):64–71.

Smith-Warner SA, Spiegelman D, Yuan SS, et al. Alcohol and breast cancer in women: a pooled analysis of cohort studies. *Journal of the American Medical Association.* 1998;279:535–540.

Smyth JM, Stone AA, Hurewitz A, and Kaell A. Effects of writing about stressful experiences on symptom reduction in patients with asthma or rheumatoid arthritis. *Journal of the American Medical Association.* 1999;281(14):1304–1309.

Spiegel D. Healing words: Emotional expression and disease outcome. *Journal of the American Medical Association.* 1999;281(14):1328–1329.

Spiegel D and Moore R. Imagery and hypnosis in the treatment of cancer patients. *Oncology.* 1997;11(8):1179–1189.

Stoll BA. Diet and exercise regimens to improve breast carcinoma prognosis. *Cancer.* 1996;78(12):2465–2470.

Stoll BA. Can unorthodox cancer therapy improve quality-of-life? *Annals of Oncology.* 1993;4(2):121–123.

Stone WL and Papas AM. Tocopherols and the etiology of colon cancer. *Journal of the National Cancer Institute.* 1997;89(14):1006–1014.

Sun AS, Ostadal O, Ryznar V, et al. Phase I/II study of stage III and IV non-small-cell lung cancer patients taking a specific dietary supplement. *Nutrition and Cancer.* 1999;34(1):62–69.

Thompson D. Acupuncture works: an NIH panel endorses the ancient needle treatment—at least for some conditions. *Time.* November 17, 1997. Page 84.

Thune I. Physical exercise in rehabilitation program for cancer patients? [commentary] *The Journal of Alternative and Complementary Medicine.* 1998;4(2):205–207.

Tokar E. Seeing to the distant mountain: diagnosis in Tibetan Medicine. *Alternative Therapies in Health and Medicine.* 1999;5(2):50–58.

Thune I, Brenn T, Lund E, and Gaard M. Physical activity and the risk of breast cancer. *New England Journal of Medicine.* 1997;336(18):1269–1275.

U.S. Congress, Office of Technology Assessment. *Unconventional Cancer Treatments.* OTA-H-405 (Washington, D.C.: U.S. Government Printing Office, September 1990).

Willett WC. Cancer prevention: diet and risk reduction. In: DeVita VT, Hellman S, and Rosenberg SA, eds. *Cancer: Principles and Practice of Oncology.* [5th edition] Philadelphia: Lippincott-Raven. 1997:559–584.

Willett WC. Diet and cancer: what do we know now? *Advances in Oncology.* 1995;11(4):3–8.

Winningham ML. Walking program for people with cancer. Getting started. *Cancer Nursing.* 199;14(5):270–276.

Yip I, Heber D, and Aronson W. Nutrition and prostate cancer. *Urologic Clinics of North America.* 1999;26(2):403–411.

Zaloznik AJ. Unproven (unorthodox) cancer treatments: a guide for healthcare professionals. *Cancer Practice.* 1994;2(1):19–24.

Chapter 7: EMOTIONAL HEALING

Derogatis LR, Morrow GR, Fetting J, et al. The prevalence of psychiatric disorders among cancer patients. *Journal of the American Medical Association.* 1983;249(6):751–757.

Fertig DL. Depression in patients with breast cancer: prevalence, diagnosis, and treatment. *The Breast Journal.* 1997;3(5):292–302.

Fox BH. The role of psychological factors in cancer incidence and prognosis. *Oncology.* 1995;9(3):245–253.

Holland JC and Breitbart W, eds. *Psychooncology.* New York: Oxford University Press. 1998.

Holland JC and Rowland JH, eds. *Handbook of Psychooncology: Psychological Care of the Patient with Cancer.* New York: Oxford University Press. 1990.

Kreitier S. Denial in cancer patients. *Cancer Investigation.* 1999;17(7):514–534.

LeShan, Lawrence, PhD. *Cancer as a Turning Point: A Handbook for People with Cancer, Their Families, and Health Professionals.* London, England: Penguin Books. 1989.

Passik SD, Dugan W, McDonald MV, et al. Oncologists' recognition of depression in their patients with cancer. *Journal of Clinical Oncology.* 1998; 16(4):1594–1600.

Pirl WF and Roth AJ. Diagnosis and treatment of depression in cancer patients. *Oncology.* 1999;13(9):1293–1301.

Smyth JM, Stone AA, Hurewitz A, and Kaell A. Effects of writing about stressful experiences on symptom reduction in patients with asthma or rheumatoid arthritis. *Journal of the American Medical Association.* 1999;281(14):1304–1309.

Spiegel D. Healing words: Emotional expression and disease outcome. *Journal of the American Medical Association.* 1999;281(14):1328–1329.

Sutor B, Rummans TA, Jowsey SG, et al. Major depression in medically ill patients. *Mayo Clinic Proceedings.* 1998;73:329–337.

Valente SM, Saunders JM, and Cohen MZ. Evaluating depression among patients with cancer. *Cancer Practice.* 1994;2(1):65–71.

CHAPTER 8: THE NATURE OF MIND

Benson H. *Timeless Healing: The Power and Biology of Belief.* New York: Scribner. 1996.

Borysenko J. *Minding the Body, Mending the Mind.* New York: Bantam Books. 1987.

Chodron T. *Taming the Monkey Mind.* Torrance, CA: Heian International, Inc. 1999.

Dossey L. *Meaning and Medicine: Lessons from a Doctor's Tales of Breakthrough and Healing.* New York: Bantam Books. 1991.

Dossey L. What does illness mean? *Alternative Therapies in Health and Medicine.* 1995;1(3):6–10.

Moyers B. *Healing and the Mind.* New York: Doubleday. 1993.

O'Connor AP, Wicker CA, and Germino BB. Understanding the cancer patient's search for meaning. *Cancer Nursing.* 1990;13:167–175.

Robbins A. *Awaken the Giant Within: How to Take Immediate Control of Your Mental, Emotional, Physical, and Financial Destiny.* New York: Summit Books. 1991.

Taylor EJ. The search for meaning among persons with cancer. *Quality of Life—A Nursing Challenge.* 1993;2(3):65–70.

CHAPTER 9: LIFE ASSESSMENT

Brown JK and Knapp TR. Do people with cancer postpone death to celebrate special occasions? *Cancer Practice.* 1995;3(6):351–355.

Frankl VE. *Man's Search for Meaning.* New York: Washington Square Press. 1985.

Hanson LC, Tulsky JA, and Danis M. Can clinical interventions change care at the end of life? *Annals of Internal Medicine.* 1997;126(5):381–388.

His Holiness the Dalai Lama. *The Meaning of Life from a Buddhist Perspective.* Translated and edited by Jeffery Hopkins. Boston: Wisdom Publications. 1992.

His Holiness the Dalai Lama and Cutler HC. *The Art of Happiness.* New York: Riverhead Books. 1998

Jones LB. *The Path: Creating Your Mission Statement for Work and for Life.* New York, NY: Hyperion. 1996.

Kübler-Ross E. *On Death and Dying: What the Dying Have to Teach Doctors, Nurses, Clergy, and Their Own Families.* New York: Touchstone. 1997.

LeShan, Lawrence, PhD. *Cancer as a Turning Point: A Handbook for People with Cancer, Their Families, and Health Professionals.* London, England: Penguin Books. 1989.

Levine S. *A Year to Live: How to Live This Year as if It Were Your Last.* New York: Bell Tower. 1997.

Levine S. *Who Dies? An Investigation of Conscious Living and Conscious Dying.* Garden City, NY: Anchor Books. 1982.

Lo B, Quill T, and Tulsky J. Discussing palliative care with patients. *Annals of Internal Medicine.* 1999;130(9):744–749.

McCarthy KW. *The On Purpose Person: Making Your Life Make Sense.* Colorado Springs, CO: Pinon Press. 1992.

McCue JD. The naturalness of dying. *Journal of the American Medical Association.* 1995;273(13):1039–1043.

Smith TJ and Schnipper LJ. The American Society of Clinical Oncology program to improve end-of-life care. *Journal of Palliative Medicine.* 1998;1(3):221–230.

Singer PA, Martin DK, and Kelner M. Quality end-of-life care: patients' perspectives. *Journal of the American Medical Association.* 1999;281(2):163–168.

Singh KD. *The Grace in Dying: How We Are Transformed Spiritually as We Die.* San Francisco: Harper. 1998.

Taylor EJ. The search for meaning among persons with cancer. *Quality of Life—A Nursing Challenge.* 1993;2(3):65–70.

Chapter 10: THE NATURE OF SPIRIT

Byrom T. *The Heart of Awareness: A Translation of the Ashtavakra Gita.* Boston: Shambhala. 1990.

Copp LA and Copp JD. Illness and the human spirit. *Quality of Life—A Nursing Challenge.* 1993;2(3):50–55.

Godman D, ed. *Be as You Are: The Teachings of Sri Ramana Maharshi.* London, England: Arkana Books. 1991.

Godman D. *Nothing Ever Happened.* Boulder, CO: Avadhuta Foundation. 1998.

Huxley A. *The Perennial Philosophy.* New York: HarperCollins. 1990.

Miller BS (translator). *The Bhagavad-Gita: Krishna's Council in Time of War.* New York: Bantam. 1986.

Nisargadatta Maharaj. *I Am That.* Bangalore, India: Nesma Books. 1997.

Poonja Sri HWL and de Jeger P, ed. *The Truth Is.* San Anselmo, CA: Vidyasagar Publishing. 1999.

Prabhavananda S and Isherwood C (translators). *Shankara's Crest-Jewel of Discrimination* (Viveka-Chudamani). Hollywood: Vedanta Press. 1978.

Rahula W. *What the Buddha Taught.* New York: Grove Press. 1962.

Smith, Huston. *The Forgotten Truth. The Common Vision of the World's Religions.* New York: HarperCollins Publishers. 1992.

Schuon, Frithjof. *The Transcendent Unity of Religions.* Wheaton, IL: Quest Books, 1993.

Venkatesananda S. *Vasistha's Yoga.* Albany, NY: State University of New York Press. 1993.

APPENDIX 1: HELPFUL BOOKS, TAPES, AND CDs

The world is full of magnificent books and other resources that can be profoundly helpful for anyone dealing with cancer or other serious illnesses. Below is a list of some of the books, tapes, and CDs that I have found over the years to be of great value for patients, family members, and friends. I have taken the liberty of categorizing the books according to the Seven-Level Program, because I have found this to be a useful way of organizing a potentially overwhelming abundance of resource materials. Please note, however, that many of these books address issues that are dealt with in more than one of the seven levels of the program. In this context, I have placed each book in what I feel is the most relevant category, and have added a supplementary list at the end containing books of general interest.

A. BOOKS

LEVEL 1: EDUCATION AND INFORMATION

General Information About Cancer

Buckman, Robert, Dr. *What You Really Need to Know About Cancer: A Comprehensive Guide for Patients and Their Families.* Baltimore: The Johns Hopkins University Press. 1997.

Dollinger, Malin, MD; Rosenbaum, Ernest, MD; and Cable, Greg. *Everyone's Guide to Cancer Therapy: How Cancer Is Diagnosed, Treated and Managed Today.* Kansas City: Andrews and McMeel. 1998.

DeVita, Vincent, Jr., MD; Hellman, Samuel, MD; and Rosenberg, Steven, MD, PhD. *Cancer: Principles and Practice of Oncology.* 5th edition. Philadelphia: Lippincott-Raven. 1997.

Schlessel-Harpham, Wendy, MD. *Diagnosis—Cancer: Your Guide Through the First Few Months.* New York: W.W. Norton & Company, Inc. 1998.

Zakarian, Beverly. *The Activist Cancer Patient: How to Take Charge of Your Treatment.* New York: John Wiley and Sons, Inc. 1996.

Weinberg, Robert A. *One Renegade Cell: How Cancer Begins.* New York: Basic Books. 1998.

Weinberg, Robert A. *Racing to the Beginning of the Road: The Search for the Origin of Cancer.* New York: W.H. Freeman and Company. 1996.

Waldholz, Michael. *Curing Cancer: Solving One of the Greatest Medical Mysteries of Our Time.* New York: Simon & Schuster. 1997.

Rosenberg, Steven A, MD, PhD, and Barry, John. *The Transformed Cell: Unlocking the Mysteries of Cancer.* New York: G. P. Putnam's Sons. 1992.

Prescott, David M., and Flexer, Abraham S. *Cancer: The Misguided Cell.* Sunderland, MA: Sinauer Associates, Inc. 1986.

Chemotherapy and Radiation

Fischer, David S.; Knobf, M. Tish; and, Durivage, Henry J. *The Cancer Chemotherapy Handbook.* St. Louis: Mosby Publishing Company. 1997.

McKay, Judith, RN, OCN, and Hirano, Nancee, RN, AOCN. *The Chemotherapy & Radiation Therapy Survival Guide: Information, Suggestions, and Support to Help You Get Through Treatment.* Oakland, CA: New Harbinger Publications, Inc. 1998.

Drum, David E. *Making the Chemotherapy Decision.* Los Angeles: Lowell House. 1996.

Bruning, Nancy Pauline. *Coping with Chemotherapy.* New York: Ballantine Books. 1993.

Drum, David E. *Making the Radiation Decision.* Los Angeles: Lowell House. 1996.

Dodd, Marylin J., RN, PhD. *Managing the Side Effects of Chemotherapy and Radiation.* New York: Prentice Hall Press. 1987.

McCollough, Virginia E. (contributor) and Cukier, Daniel. *Coping with Radiation Therapy: A Ray of Hope.* Baltimore: Contemporary Books. 1996.

Breast Cancer

Link, John, MD. *The Breast Cancer Survival Manual: A Step-by-Step Guide for the Woman With Newly Diagnosed Breast Cancer.* New York: Henry Holt and Company, Inc. 1998.

Austin, Steve, MD, and Hitchcock, Cathy, MSW. *Breast Cancer: What You Should Know (But May Not Be Told) About Prevention, Diagnosis, and Treatment.* Rocklin, CA: Prima Publishing. 1994.

Swirsky, Joan, and Balaban, Barbara. *The Breast Cancer Handbook: Taking Control After You've Found a Lump.* New York: HarperCollins. 1994.

Brinker, Nancy. *The Race Is Run One Step at a Time: Everywoman's Guide.* New York: Simon & Schuster. 1990.

Love, Susan M., MD. *Dr. Susan Love's Breast Book.* Reading, MA: Addison-Wesley Publishing Company. 1990.

Mayer, Musa. *Holding Tight, Letting Go: Living with Metastatic Breast Cancer.* Sebastopol, CA: O'Reilly & Associates. 1997.

Stabiner, Karen. *To Dance with the Devil: The New War On Breast Cancer—Politics, Power, and People.* New York: Delacorte Press. 1997.

Prostate Cancer

Morra, Marion E.; Potts, Eve (contributor); Muinos, Hilda R. (illustrator); and DeVita, Vincent, MD. *The Prostate Cancer Answer Book: An Unbiased Guide to Treatment Choices.* New York: Avon Books. 1996.

Kirby, Roger S.; Christmas, Timothy J.; and Brawer, Michael. *Prostate Cancer.* New York: Times Mirror International Publishers Limited. 1996.

Walsh, Patrick C., MD, and Worthington, Janet Farrar (contributor). *The Prostate: A Guide for Men and the Women Who Love Them.* New York: Warner Books. 1997.

Rous, Stephen N., MD. *The Prostate Book: Sound Advice on Symptoms and Treatment.* New York: W.W. Norton & Co. 1994.

Salcedo, H., MD, FACS. *The Prostate: Facts and Misconceptions.* Secaucus, NJ: Birch Lane Press. 1993.

Korda, Michael. *Man to Man: Surviving Prostate Cancer.* New York: Vintage Books. 1997.

Garnick, Marc B. *The Patient's Guide to Prostate Cancer: An Expert's Successful Treatment Strategies and Options.* New York: Plume Publishers. 1996.

Lung Cancer

Cox, Barbara G.; Carr, David T.; Harmon, Eloise; and Lee, Robert E. *Living with Lung Cancer: A Guide for Patients and Their Families.* Gainesville, FL: Triad Publishing Company. 1998.

Ruckdeschel, John C., MD. *Myths & Facts About Lung Cancer.* Philadelphia: W. B. Saunders Company. 1999.

Peters, Tim. *A Patient Guide to COPD & Lung Cancer.* Peapack, NJ: Humanatomy Board Books. 1991.

Colon Cancer

Miskovitz, Paul, MD. *What to Do If You Get Colon Cancer: A Specialist Helps You Take Charge and Make Informed Choices.* New York: John Wiley & Sons, Inc. 1997.

Pazdur, Richard, MD, and Royce, Melanie, MD. *Myths & Facts about Colorectal Cancer.* Melville, NY: PRR. 1998.

Levin, Bernard, MD. *The American Cancer Society: Colorectal Cancer.* New York: Random House. 1999.

Ovarian Cancer

Piver, M. Steven, MD, and Wilder, Gene (contributor). *Gilda's Disease: Sharing Personal Experiences and a Medical Perspective on Ovarian Cancer.* New York: Broadway Books. 1998.

Piver, M. Steven, MD, and Eltabbakh, Gamal, MD. *Myths & Facts About Ovarian Cancer.* Melville, NY: PRR. 1997.

Tilberis, Liz. *No Time to Die: Living with Ovarian Cancer.* New York: Avon Books. 1999.

Lymphoma

Johnston, Lorraine, and Lamb, Linda. *Non-Hodgkin's Lymphomas: Making Sense of Diagnosis, Treatment, and Options.* Sebastopol, CA: O'Reilly & Associates. 1999.

Canellos, George P.; Lister, T.A.; Sklar, Jeffrey L.; and Lampert, Richard (editors). *The Lymphomas.* Philadelphia: W. B. Saunders Company. 1998.

Mauch, Peter M.; Armitage, James O.; Diehl, Volker; Hoppe, Richard T.; and Weiss, Lawrence M. (editors). *Hodgkin's Disease.* Philadelphia: Lippincott Williams & Wilkins. 1999.

LEVEL 2: PSYCHOSOCIAL SUPPORT

Spiegel, David, MD. *Living Beyond Limits: New Hope and Help for Facing Life-Threatening Illness.* New York: Random House. 1993.

Ornish, Dean, MD. *Love & Survival: The Scientific Basis for the Healing Power of Intimacy.* New York: HarperCollins Publishers, Inc. 1998.

Benjamin, Harold, PhD. *From Victim to Victor: The Wellness Community Guide to Fighting for Recovery for Cancer Patients and Their Families.* Los Angeles: Jeremy P. Tarcher, Inc. 1987.

McFarland, John Robert. *Now That I Have Cancer...I Am Whole: Meditations for Cancer Patients and Those Who Love Them.* Kansas City: Andrews and McMeel. 1993.

Carter, Rosalynn. *Helping Yourself Help Others: A Book for Caregivers.* New York: Random House. 1994.

Anderson, Greg. *The Cancer Conqueror: An Incredible Journey to Wellness.* Kansas City: Andrews and McMeel. 1988.

Edge, Fred. *Borrowed Time: Living with Cancer with Someone You Love.* Lantzville, British Columbia, Canada: Oolichan Books. 1995.

LEVEL 3: THE BODY AS GARDEN

Complementary and Alternative Cancer Treatments

Lerner, Michael, PhD. *Choices in Healing: Integrating the Best of Conventional and Complementary Approaches to Cancer.* Cambridge, MA: The MIT Press. 1994.

Pelton, Ross, RPH, PhD, and Overholser, Lee, PhD. *Alternatives in Cancer Therapy: The Complete Guide to Non-Traditional Treatments.* New York: Fireside. 1994.

Walters, Richard. *Options, The Alternative Cancer Therapy Book: For People Who Want to Make Informed Decisions About Alternative Cancer Treatments.* Garden City, NY: Avery Publishing Group, Inc. 1993.

Cassileth, Barrie R., PhD. *The Alternative Medicine Handbook: The Complete Reference Guide to Alternative and Complementary Therapies.* New York: W. W. Norton & Company. 1998.

Diamond, W. John, MD, and Cowden, Lee, MD, with Goldberg, Burton. *Definitive Guide to Alternative Medicine.* Tiburon, CA: Future Medicine Publishing, Inc. 1997.

Moss, Ralph W., PhD. *Herbs Against Cancer: History and Controversy.* Brooklyn: Equinox Press, Inc. 1998.

Moss, Ralph W., PhD. *Cancer Therapy: The Independent Consumer's Guide to Non-Toxic Treatment & Prevention.* New York: Equinox Press. 1992.

Boik, John. *Cancer and Natural Medicine: A Textbook of Basic Science and Clinical Research.* Princeton, MN: Oregon Medical Press. 1996.

Hartwell, Jonathan L. *Plants Used Against Cancer.* Lawrence, MA: Quarterman Publications, Inc. 1982.

Diet and Nutrition

Spiller, Gene, PhD, and Bruce, Bonnie, MD, PhD, RD. *Cancer Survivor's Nutrition and Health Guide: Eating Well and Getting Better During and After Cancer Treatment.* Rocklin, CA: Prima Publishing. 1997.

Quillin, Patrick, PhD, RD. *Beating Cancer with Nutrition: Clinically Proven and Easy-to-Follow Strategies to Dramatically Improve Your Quality of Life and Chances for a Complete Remission.* Tulsa, OK: The Nutrition Times Press, Inc. 1994.

Keane, Maureen; Chace, Daniella (contributor); and Lung, John A. *What to Eat If You Have Cancer: A Guide to Adding Nutritional Therapy to Your Treatment Plan.* Lincolnwood, IL: NTC/Contemporary Publishing. 1996.

Calhoun, Susan, et al. *Nutrition, Cancer and You: What You Need to Know, and Where to Start.* Lenexa, KS: Addax Publishing Group. 1997.

Robbins, John. *Diet for a New America: How Your Food Choices Affect Your Health, Happiness and the Future of Life on Earth.* Walpole, NH: Stillpoint Publishing. 1987.

Diamond, Harvey; Diamond, Marilyn; and Lawrence, Kay S. *Fit for Life*. New York: Warner Books. 1987.

Murray, Michael T., ND. *The Healing Power of Foods: Nutrition Secrets for Vibrant Health and Long Life*. Rocklin, CA: Prima Publishing. 1993.

Binzel, Jr., Philip E., MD. *Alive and Well: One Doctor's Experience with Nutrition in the Treatment of Cancer Patients*. Westlake Village, CA: American Media. 1994.

Griffiths, K.; Adlercreutz, H.; Boyle, P.; Denis, L.; Nicholson, R.I.; and Morton, M.S. *Nutrition and Cancer*. Oxford, UK: ISIS Medical Media. 1996.

Kushi, Michio, and Esko, Edward. *The Macrobiotic Approach to Cancer: Toward Preventing and Controlling Cancer with Diet and Lifestyle*. Garden City, NY: Avery Publishing Group. 1991.

Cousens, Gabriel, MD. *Spiritual Nutrition and the Rainbow Diet*. Boulder, CO: Cassandra Press. 1986.

Herbs and Supplements

Griffith, H. Winter. *Vitamins, Herbs, Minerals & Supplements: The Complete Guide*. New York: Fine Communications. 1999.

Alive Books Staff (editor). *The All in One Guide to Herbs, Vitamins & Minerals: The Quick and Easy Reference for Everything You Need to Know*. Blaine, WA: Alive Books. 1998.

Navarra, Tova (editor); Navarra, John G.; and Lipkowitz, Myron A. *Encyclopedia of Vitamins, Minerals and Supplements*. New York: Facts On File, Inc. 1997.

Bown, Deni. *Encyclopedia of Herbs & Their Uses*. New York: Ingram Publishing. 1995.

Murray, Michael T. *Encyclopedia of Nutritional Supplements: The Essential Guide for Improving Your Health Naturally*. Rocklin, CA: Prima Publishing. 1996.

Weiner, Michael A., and Weiner, Janet A. *Herbs That Heal, RX: Prescription for Herbal Healing*. Mill Valley, CA: Quantum Books. 1994.

Santillo, Humbart N.D. *Natural Healing with Herbs: The Complete Reference Book for the Use of Herbs*. Prescott, AZ: Hohm Press. 1993.

Tyler, Varro E., PhD. *The New Honest Herbal: A Sensible Guide to Herbs and Related Remedies*. Philadelphia: George F. Stickley Company. 1987.

Bremness, Lesley. *The Complete Book of Herbs*. Bergenfield, NJ: Studio Books. 1988.

Frawley, David, Dr., and Lad, Vasant, Dr. *The Yoga of Herbs: An Ayurvedic Guide to Herbal Medicine*. Santa Fe: Lotus Press. 1986.

Aromatherapy

Schnaubelt, Kurt. *Advanced Aromatherapy: The Science of Essential Oil Therapy*. Rochester, VT: Inner Traditions International Limited. 1998.

Lawless, Julia. *The Complete Illustrated Guide to Aromatherapy: A Practical Approach to the Use of Essential Oils for Health and Well-Being*. Boston: Element Books. 1997.

Wildwood, Christine. *The Encyclopedia of Aromatherapy*. Rochester, VT: Inner Traditions International Limited. 1996.

Exercise

Andes, Karen. *The Complete Book of Fitness: Mind, Body, Spirit*. New York: Fitness Magazine. Three Rivers Press. 1999.

Reichler, Gayle, and Burke, Nancy. *Active Wellness: A Personalized 10 Step Program for a Healthy Body, Mind & Spirit*. Alexandria, VA: Time Life, Inc. 1998.

Cooper, Kenneth H., MD. *The Aerobics Program for Total Well-Being: Exercise, Diet, Emotional Balance*. New York: Bantam/Doubleday/Dell Publishing Company. 1985.

Kilham, Christopher S. *The Five Tibetans: Five Dynamic Exercises for Health, Energy and Personal Power*. Rochester, NY: Inner Traditions International Limited. 1994.

Feldenkrais, Moshe. *Awareness Through Movement: Health Exercises for Personal Growth*. San Francisco: HarperSanFrancisco. 1991.

Kelder, Peter (editor), and Siegel, Bernie S. *Ancient Secret of the Fountain of Youth*. New York: Doubleday. 1998.

Farhi, Donna. *The Breathing Book: Vitality & Good Health Through Essential Breath Work*. New York: Henry Holt & Company, Inc. 1995.

Zi, Nancy. *The Art of Breathing: Six Simple Lessons to Improve Performance, Health & Well-Being*. Glendale, CA: VIVI Company. 1997.

Hendricks, Gay. *Conscious Breathing: Breathwork for Health, Stress Release, and Personal Mastery*. New York: Ingram Publishing. 1997.

Yoga

Feuerstein, Georg. *The Shambhala Guide to Yoga: An Essential Introduction to the Principles and Practice of an Ancient Tradition*. Boston: Shambhala Publications, Inc. 1996.

Pierce, Margaret D., and Pierce, Martin G. *Yoga for Your Life: A Practice Manual of Breath and Movement for Every Body*. Portland, OR: Rudra Press. 1996.

Satchidananda, Sri Swami. *Integral Yoga Hatha*. Buckingham, VA: Integral Yoga Distribution. 1998.

Vishnudevananda, Swami. *The Complete Illustrated Book of Yoga*. New York: Crown Publishers. 1995.

Iyengar, B.K.S., and Menuhin, Yeudi. *Light on Yoga: Yoga Dipika*. New York: Schocken Books. 1995.

Christensen, Alice. *The American Yoga Association Wellness Book*. New York: Kensington Publications Corp. 1996.

Sarley, Dinabandhu, and Sarley, Ila. *The Essentials of Yoga*. New York: Dell. 1999.

Relaxation

Blumenfield, Larry (editor); Gawain, Shakti; and Folan, Lilias (contributor). *The Big Book of Relaxation: Simple Techniques to Control the Excess Stress in Your Life.* Roslyn, NY: Relaxation Company. 1994.

Lacroix, Nitya, and Bown, Deni. *101 Essential Tips: Relaxation.* New York: DK Publishing Merchandise. 1998.

Davis, Martha; Eshelman, Elizabeth Robbins; and McKay, Matthew. *Relaxation & Stress Reduction Workbook.* Upland, PA: Diane Publishing Company. 1997.

Sutcliffe, Jenny. *The Complete Book of Relaxation Techniques.* Allentown, PA: Peoples Medical Society. 1994.

George, Mike. *Learn to Relax: A Practical Guide to Easing Tension and Conquering Stress.* San Francisco: Chronicle Books. 1998.

Benson, Herbert, MD, and Klipper, Miriam Z. *The Relaxation Response.* New York: Avon Books. 1990.

Massage

Mumford, Susan. *Healing Massage: A Practical Guide to Relaxation and Well-Being.* New York: Plume. 1998.

Mitchell, Stewart. *The Complete Illustrated Guide to Massage: A Step-by-Step Approach to the Healing Art of Touch.* Boston: Element Books, Inc. 1997.

Ruhnke, Amiyo. *Body Wisdom: Simple Massage and Relaxation Techniques for Busy People.* New York: Tuttle Books, Inc. 1996.

Maxwell-Hudson, Clare. *The Complete Book of Massage.* New York: Random House. 1998.

Lidell, Lucinda. *The Book of Massage: The Complete Step-by-Step Guide to Eastern and Western Techniques.* New York: Simon & Schuster. 1984.

Porter, Sarah. *Massage: For Health, Relaxation and Vitality.* New York: Lorenz Books. 1998.

MacDonald, Gayle. *Medicine Hands: Massage Therapy for People with Cancer.* Portland, OR: Rudra Press. 1999.

Journaling

Gullo, Shirley. *Journaling Through the Storm: A Journal for Personal Reflections.* Pittsburgh: Oncology Nursing Society. 1998.

Neimark, Neil F., MD. *The Handbook of Journaling: Tools for the Healing of Mind, Body & Spirit.* R.E.P. Technologies. 1998.

Forrest, Jan. *Coming Home to Ourselves: Journaling to Wholeness.* West Olive, MI: Heart to Heart. 1998.

Hossler, Bill. *Keys to Open Your Heart: A Journaling Guide for Men and Women.* Bakersfield, CA: Key Publications. 1998.

DeSalvo, Louise, PhD. *Writing as a Way of Healing.* San Francisco: HarperSan-Francisco. 1999.

Guarino, Lois. *Writing Your Authentic Self.* New York: Dell. 1999.

Visualization and Guided Imagery

Naparstek, Belleruth. *Staying Well with Guided Imagery: How to Harness the Power of Your Imagination for Health and Healing.* New York: Warner Books, Inc. 1994.

Gawain, Shakti. *Creative Visualization.* New York: Bantam Books. 1983.

Fanning, Patrick. *Visualization for Change: A Step-by-Step Guide to Using the Powers of Your Imagination for Self-improvement, Therapy, Healing, and Pain Control.* Oakland, CA: New Harbinger. 1988.

Achterberg, Jeanne, PhD; Dossey, Barbara, RN, MS, FAAN; and Kolkmeier, Leslie, RN, MEd. *Rituals of Healing: Using Imagery for Health and Wellness.* New York: Bantam New Age Books. 1994.

Brigham, Deirdre Davis. *Imagery for Getting Well: Clinical Applications of Behavioral Medicine.* New York: W. W. Norton & Company, Inc. 1994.

Lusk, Julie T. *Thirty Scripts for Relaxation Imagery & Inner Healing, Volume 2.* Duluth, MN: Whole Person Associates, Inc. 1993.

Acupuncture

Nightingale, Michael. *Acupuncture: An Introductory Guide to the Technique and Its Benefits.* North Pomfret, VT: Trafalgar Square. 1997.

Mole, Peter. *Acupuncture: Energy Balancing for Body, Mind and Spirit ("Health Essentials" Series).* Boston: Element Books, Inc. 1997.

Firebrace, Peter. *Acupuncture: How It Works, How It Cures.* Lincolnwood, IL: NTC/Contemporary Publishing Company. 1994.

Chang, Stephen Thomas. *The Complete Book of Acupuncture.* Berkeley: Celestial Arts Publishing Company. 1983.

Chiropractic

Dahlin, Donald A. *Chiropractic for Natural Health and Wellness Care.* Chicago: Adams Press. 1993.

Burke, Edmund J., and Gravelle, Brent L. *Wellness and Chiropractic.* Longmeadow, MA: Mouvement Publications. 1997.

Redwood, Daniel. *Contemporary Chiropractic.* New York: Churchill Livingstone, Inc. 1997.

McGill, Leonard. *The Chiropractor's Health Book: Simple, Natural Exercises for Relieving Headaches, Tension, and Back Pain.* New York: Crown Publishers. 1997.

Rondberg, Terry A. *Chiropractic First: The Fastest Growing Healthcare Choice Before Drugs or Surgery.* Chandler, AZ: The Chiropractic Journal. 1996.

Koch, William H. *Chiropractic: The Superior Alternative*. Nashville, TN: Associated Publishers. 1997.

Homeopathy

Hammond, Christopher. *The Complete Family Guide to Homeopathy: An Illustrated Encyclopedia of Safe and Effective Remedies*. New York: Viking Penguin. 1996.

Vithoulkas, George, and Tiller, William A. *Science of Homeopathy*. New York: Grove Atlantic, Inc. 1980.

Jonas, Wayne B., and Jacobs, Jennifer. *Healing with Homeopathy: The Complete Guide*. New York: Warner Books, Inc. 1996.

Weiner, Michael. *The Complete Book of Homeopathy*. Garden City, NY: Avery Publishing Group, Inc. 1989.

Bruning, Nancy Pauling, and Sonberg, Lynn. *Healing Homeopathic Remedies*. New York: Dell. 1996.

Therapeutic Touch

Krieger, Dolores. *Accepting Your Power to Heal: The Personal Practice of Therapeutic Touch*. Santa Fe, NM: Bear & Company. 1993.

Krieger, Dolores. *The Therapeutic Touch: How to Use Your Hands to Help to Heal*. Indianapolis: Simon & Schuster/Macmillan General Reference. 1992.

Cowens, Deborah, and Monte, Tom. *A Gift for Healing: How You Can Use Therapeutic Touch*. New York: Crown Publishers. 1996.

MacRae, Janet. *Therapeutic Touch: A Practical Guide*. New York: Alfred A. Knopf, Inc. 1988.

Reiki Therapy

Parkes, Chris. *Reiki: The Essential Guide to the Ancient Healing Art*. Freedom, CA: The Crossing Press, Inc. 1999.

Shuffey, Sandi Leir. *Reiki: A Beginner's Guide*. London, England: Hodder and Stoughton. 1998.

Lubeck, Walter. *The Complete Reiki Handbook: Basic Introduction and Methods of Natural Application, a Complete Guide for Reiki Practice*. Twin Lakes, WI: Lotus Light Publications. 1998.

Stein, Diane. *Essential Reiki: A Complete Guide to an Ancient Healing Art*. Freedom, CA: The Crossing Press. 1995.

Honervoght, Tanmaya. *The Power of Reiki: An Ancient Hands-On Healing Technique*. New York: Henry Holt & Company. 1998.

Upczak, Patrick Rose. *Reiki: A Way of Life*. Nederland, CO: Synchronicity Publishing. 1999.

Horan, Paula. *Empowerment Through Reiki: Path to Personal and Global Transformation*. Twin Lakes, WI: Lotus Light Publications. 1998.

EASTERN HEALING TRADITIONS

Ayurveda

Tiwari, Maya. *Ayurveda Secrets of Healing: The Complete Ayurvedic Guide to Healing Through Pancha Karma Seasonal Therapies, Diet, Herbal Remedies and Memory.* Twin Lakes, WI: Lotus Press. 1995.

Lad, Vasant, Dr. *Ayurveda: The Science of Self-Healing.* Santa Fe, NM: Lotus Press. 1984.

Morrison, Judith H. *The Book of Ayurveda: A Holistic Approach to Health and Longevity.* New York: Simon & Schuster. 1995.

Frawley, David, Dr. *Ayurvedic Healing: A Comprehensive Guide.* Salt Lake City: Passage Press. 1989.

Frawley, David, Dr. *Ayurveda and the Mind: the Healing of Consciousness.* Twin Lakes, WI: Lotus Press. 1996.

Joshi, Sunil V. V., Dr. *Ayurveda and Panchakarma: The Science of Healing and Rejuvenation.* Twin Lakes, WI: Lotus Light Publications. 1997.

Warrier, Gopi, and Bunawant, Deepika. *The Complete Illustrated Guide to Ayurveda: The Ancient Indian Healing Tradition.* Boston: Element Books. 1997.

Traditional Chinese Medicine

Beinfeld, Harriet, and Corngold, Efrom. *Between Heaven and Earth: A Guide to Chinese Medicine.* New York: Ballantine. 1992.

Williams, Tom. *Chinese Medicine, Acupuncture, Herbal Remedies, Nutrition, Qigong and Meditation for Total Health.* Boston: Element Books, Inc. 1998.

Kaptchuk, Ted J., OMD. *The Web That Has No Weaver: Understanding Chinese Medicine.* New York: Congdon and Weed. 1983.

Kun, Jia. *Prevention and Treatment of Carcinoma in Traditional Chinese Medicine.* Hong Kong: The Commercial Press, Ltd. 1985.

Leung, Albert Y. *Chinese Herbal Remedies.* New York: Universe Books. 1984.

Tibetan Medicine

Donden, Yeshi, Dr. *Health Through Balance: An Introduction to Tibetan Medicine.* Ithaca, NY: Snow Lion Publications. 1986.

Donden, Yeshi, and Kelsang, Jhampa (translator). *The Ambrosia Heart Tantra: The Secret Oral Teaching on the Eight Branches of the Science of Healing.* Dharamsala, India: Library of Tibetan Works and Archives. 1995.

Clifford, Terry. *Tibetan Buddhist Medicine and Psychiatry: The Diamond Healing.* York Beach, ME: Samuel Weiser, Inc. 1984.

Clark, Barry, Dr. (translator). *The Quintessence Tantras of Tibetan Medicine.* Ithaca, NY: Snow Lion Publications, Inc. 1995.

Finckh, Elisabeth. *Foundations of Tibetan Medicine, According to the Book rGyud bzi. Volume One.* London, England: Robinson and Watkins Books, Ltd. 1978.

Finckh, Elisabeth. *Foundations of Tibetan Medicine, According to the Book rGyud bzi. Volume Two.* Longmead, England: Element Books, Ltd. 1988.

Dummer, Tom. *Tibetan Medicine, and Other Holistic Health-Care Systems.* London: Routledge. 1988.

Fenton, Peter. *Tibetan Healing. The Modern Legacy of Medicine Buddha.* Wheaton, IL: Quest Books, 1999.

Aschoff, Jürgen C., and Rösing, Ina (editors). *Tibetan Medicine. East Meets West— West Meets East.* Ulm, Germany: Fabri Verlag. 1997.

Chang, Garma C. C. *Teachings of Tibetan Yoga: An Introduction to the Spiritual, Mental, and Physical Exercises of the Tibetan Religion.* Secaucus, NJ: Citadel Press. 1993.

Avedon, John F. (editor). *The Buddha's Art of Healing: Tibetan Paintings Rediscovered.* New York: Rizzoli Bookstore/Arthur M. Sackler Gallery. 1998.

Parfionovitch, Yuri (editor). *Tibetan Medical Paintings: Illustrations to the Blue Beryl Treatise of Sangye Gyamtso (1653-1705: Plates and Text).* St. Louis, MO: Mosby-Year Book, Inc. 1992.

Level 4: Emotional Healing

Pennebaker, James W., PhD. *Opening Up: The Healing Power of Expressing Emotions.* New York: The Guilford Press. 1990.

Borysenko, Joan, PhD. *Guilt Is the Teacher, Love Is the Lesson: A Book to Heal You, Heart and Soul.* New York: Warner Books. 1990.

Jampolski, Gerald G., MD. *Love Is Letting Go of Fear.* Berkeley: Celestial Arts. 1979.

Jampolski, Gerald G., MD. *Teach Only Love: The Seven Principles of Attitudinal Healing.* New York: Bantam Books. 1983.

Jampolski, Gerald G., MD. *Out of Darkness into the Light: A Journey of Inner Healing.* New York: Bantam Books. 1990.

Bradshaw, John. *Healing the Shame That Binds You.* Deerfield Beach, FL: Health Communications, Inc. 1988.

Bradshaw, John. *Home Coming: Reclaiming and Championing Your Inner Child.* New York: Bantam Books. 1990.

Kurtz, Ron. *Body-Centered Psychotherapy: The Hakomi Method.* Mendocino, CA: Life Rhythm. 1990.

Zweig, Connie, PhD, and Wolf, Steve, PhD. *Romancing the Shadow: Illuminating the Dark Side of the Soul.* New York: Ballantine Books. 1997.

LEVEL 5: THE NATURE OF MIND

Moyers, Bill. *Healing and the Mind.* New York: Doubleday. 1993.

Dossey, Larry, MD. *Meaning and Medicine: Lessons from a Doctor's Tales of Breakthrough and Healing.* New York: Bantam Books. 1991.

Benson, Herbert, MD. *Timeless Healing: The Power and Biology of Belief.* New York: Scribner. 1996.

Chodron, Thubten. *Taming the Monkey Mind.* Torrance, CA: Heian International, Inc. 1999.

Borysenko, Joan, PhD. *Minding the Body, Mending the Mind.* New York: Bantam Books. 1987.

Pelletier, Kenneth R. *Mind as Healer; Mind as Slayer: A Holistic Approach to Preventing Stress Disorders.* New York: Dell. 1977.

Thondup, Tulku. *The Healing Power of Mind: Simple Meditation Exercises for Health, Well-Being, and Enlightenment.* Boston: Shambhala Publications. 1996.

Robbins, Anthony. *Awaken the Giant Within: How to Take Immediate Control of Your Mental, Emotional, Physical, and Financial Destiny.* New York: Summit Books. 1991.

Allen, James. *As a Man Thinketh.* New York: Grosset and Dunlap. 1983.

Doyle, Bruce I., III. *Before You Think Another Thought. An Illustrated Guide to Understanding How Your Thoughts and Beliefs Create Your Life.* Charlottesville, VA: Hampton Roads Publishing Company, Inc. 1997.

Jampolsky, Gerald G., MD, and Cirincione, Diane V. *Change Your Mind, Change Your Life.* New York: Bantam Books. 1994.

Roger, John, and McWilliams, Peter. *You Can't Afford the Luxury of a Negative Thought: A Book for People with Any Life-threatening Illness—Including Life.* Los Angeles: Prelude Press, Inc. 1988.

LEVEL 6: LIFE ASSESSMENT

Purpose, Mission, and Vision

Jones, Laurie Beth. *The Path: Creating Your Mission Statement for Work and for Life.* New York: Hyperion. 1996.

McCarthy, Kevin W. *The On Purpose Person: Making Your Life Make Sense.* Colorado Springs, CO: Pinon Press. 1992.

Levine, Stephen. *A Year to Live: How to Live This Year as if It Were Your Last.* New York: Bell Tower. 1997.

Bellamy, D. Richard, Dr. *12 Secrets for Manifesting Your Vision, Inspiration, and Purpose: How to Make Your Dreams Come True.* Houston, TX: PHI Publishing. 1999.

Ardell, Donald B., PhD. *The Book of Wellness: A Secular Approach to Spirituality, Meaning & Purpose.* Amherst, NY: Prometheus Books. 1996.

Covey, Stephen R. *First Things First.* New York: Simon & Schuster. 1994.

Frankl, Victor E. *Man's Search for Meaning.* New York: Washington Square Press. 1985.

Hansen, Mark Victor. *Future Diary.* Newport Beach, CA: Mark Victor Hansen Publishing Co. 1994.

Letting Go: Death and Dying

Albom, Mitch. *Tuesdays with Morrie: An Old Man, A Young Man, and Life's Greatest Lesson.* New York: Doubleday. 1997.

Levine, Stephen. *Who Dies? An Investigation of Conscious Living and Conscious Dying.* Garden City, NY: Anchor Books. 1982.

Longaker, Christine. *Facing Death and Finding Hope: A Guide to the Emotional and Spiritual Care of the Dying.* New York: Doubleday. 1997.

Tobin, Daniel R., MD, with Lindsey, Karen. *Peaceful Dying: The Step-by-Step Guide to Preserving Your Dignity, Your Choice, and Your Inner Peace at the End of Life.* Reading, MA: Perseus Books. 1999.

Singh, Kathleen Dowling. *The Grace in Dying: How We Are Transformed Spiritually as We Die.* San Francisco: HarperCollins. 1998.

Kübler-Ross, Elisabeth, MD. *On Death and Dying: What the Dying Have to Teach Doctors, Nurses, Clergy, and Their Own Families.* New York: Touchstone. 1997.

Mullin, Glenn H. *Living in the Face of Death: The Tibetan Tradition.* Ithaca, NY: Snow Lion Publications. 1998.

Byock, Ira, MD. *Dying Well. Peace and Possibilities at the End of Life.* New York: Riverhead Books. 1997.

LEVEL 7: THE NATURE OF SPIRIT

Godman, David (editor). *Be as You Are: The Teachings of Sri Ramana Maharshi.* London, England: Arkana Books. 1991.

Godman, David. *Nothing Ever Happened.* Boulder, CO: Avadhuta Foundation. 1998.

Poonja, Sri H.W.L., and de Jeger, Prashanti (editor). *The Truth Is.* San Anselmo, CA: Vidyasagar Publishing. 1999.

Poonja, Sri H.W.L.; de Jeger, Prashanti; Vidyavati and Yudhishtara (compilers and editors) *This. Prose and Poetry of Dancing Emptiness.* San Anselmo, CA: Vidyasagar Publishing. 1997.

Nisargadatta Maharaj. *I Am That.* Bangalore, India: Nesma Books. 1997.

Ardagh, Arjuna Nick. *Relaxing into Clear Seeing*. San Rafael, CA: Self Xpress. 1998.

Huxley, Aldous. *The Perennial Philosophy*. New York: HarperCollins. 1990.

Rinpoche, Sogyal. *The Tibetan Book of Living and Dying*. New York: Harper-Collins. 1994.

Goleman, Daniel, PhD, and Tarcher, J.P. *The Meditative Mind*. New York: The Putnam Publishing Group. 1988.

Kabat-Zinn, Jon, PhD. *Wherever You Go, There You Are*. New York: Hyperion/St. Martin's Press, Inc. 1994.

Kabat-Zinn, Jon, PhD. *Full Catastrophe Living: Using the Wisdom of Your Body and Mind to Face Stress, Pain, and Illness*. New York: Delta. 1990.

Dossey, Larry, MD. *Healing Words: The Power of Prayer and the Practice of Medicine*. New York: HarperCollins. 1993.

Dossey, Larry, MD. *Prayer Is Good Medicine: How to Reap the Healing Benefits of Prayer*. New York: HarperCollins. 1996.

His Holiness the Dalai Lama. *The Meaning of Life from a Buddhist Perspective*. Translated and edited by Jeffery Hopkins. Boston: Wisdom Publications. 1992.

His Holiness the Dalai Lama and Cutler, Howard, MD. *The Art of Happiness: A Handbook for Living*. New York: Riverhead Books. 1998.

Rahula, Walpola. *What the Buddha Taught*. New York: Grove Press. 1962.

Evans-Wentz, Walter Yeeling (editor). *The Tibetan Book of the Great Liberation*. New York: Oxford University Press. 1983.

Thurman, Robert A.F. (translator). *The Tibetan Book of the Dead*. New York: Bantam Books. 1994.

Garfield, Jay L. (translation and commentary). *The Fundamental Wisdom of the Middle Way: Nagarjuna's Mulamadhyamakakarika*. New York: Oxford University Press. 1995.

Smith, Huston. *The World's Religions*. New York: HarperCollins. 1991.

Smith, Huston. *The Forgotten Truth. The Common Vision of the World's Religions*. New York: HarperCollins. 1992.

Schuon, Frithjof. *The Transcendent Unity of Religions*. Wheaton, IL: Quest Books. 1993.

Levine, Stephen. *A Gradual Awakening*. Garden City, NY: Anchor Press/Double-day. 1979.

Miller, Barabara Stoler (translator). *The Bhagavad-Gita: Krishna's Council in Time of War*. New York: Bantam. 1986.

Byrom, Thomas. *The Heart of Awareness: A Translation of the Ashtavakra Gita*. Boston: Shambhala. 1990.

Venkatesananda, Swami. *Vasistha's Yoga*. Albany, NY: State University of New York Press. 1993.

Prabhavananda, Swami, and Isherwood, Christopher (translators). *Shankara's Crest-Jewel of Discrimination* (Viveka-Chudamani). Hollywood: Vedanta Press. 1978.

Zukav, Gary. *The Seat of the Soul.* New York: Fireside. 1990

OTHER HELPFUL BOOKS

Simon, David, MD. *Return to Wholeness: Embracing Body, Mind, and Spirit in the Face of Cancer.* New York: John Wiley & Sons, Inc. 1999.

Simon, David, MD. *The Wisdom of Healing: A Natural Mind Body Program for Optimal Wellness.* New York: Harmony Books. 1997.

Cousins, Norman. *Head First: The Biology of Hope.* New York: E. P. Dutton. 1989.

Cousins, Norman. *Anatomy of an Illness as Perceived by the Patient.* New York: Bantam Books. 1991.

Gordon, James S., MD. *Manifesto for a New Medicine.* Reading, MA: Addison-Wesley Publishing Company, Inc. 1996.

Gaynor, Mitchell, MD. *Healing Essence: A Cancer Doctor's Practical Program for Hope and Recovery.* New York: Kodansha America, Inc. 1995.

Gaynor, Mitchell, MD. *Sounds of Healing: A Physician Reveals the Therapeutic Power of Sound, Voice, and Music.* New York: Broadway Books. 1999.

Pert, Candace B., PhD. *Molecules of Emotion: Why You Feel the Way You Feel.* New York: Scribner. 1997.

Remen, Rachel Naomi, MD. *Kitchen Table Wisdom: Stories That Heal.* New York: Riverhead Books. 1996.

LeShan, Lawrence, PhD. *Cancer as a Turning Point: A Handbook for People with Cancer, Their Families, and Health Professionals.* London, England: Penguin Books. 1989.

Siegel, Bernie, MD. *Love, Medicine, and Miracles: Lessons Learned About Self-Healing from a Surgeon's Experience with Exceptional Patients.* New York: HarperCollins. 1986.

Simonton, O. Carl, MD. *Getting Well Again.* New York: Bantam Books. 1992.

Cunningham, Alastair J., PhD. *The Healing Journey, Overcoming the Crisis of Cancer.* Toronto, Ontario, Canada: Key Porter Books Limited. 1992.

Warner, Gale; Kreger, David; and Siegel, Bernie S., MD. *Dancing at the Edge of Life: A Memoir.* New York: Hyperion. 1998.

Ryder, Brent G. *The Alpha Book on Cancer and Living.* Alameda, CA: The Alpha Institute. 1993.

Walsch, Neale Donald. *Conversations with God: An Uncommon Dialogue, Volumes 1-3.* New York: G. P. Putnam's Sons. 1996.

Rodegast, Pat. *Emmanuel's Book: A Manual for Living Comfortably in the Cosmos, Volumes 1-3*. New York: Bantam Books. 1985.

Schulz, Mona Lisa, MD, PhD. *Awakening Intuition: Using Your Mind-Body Network for Insight and Healing*. New York: Harmony Books. 1998.

Chopra, Deepak, MD. *Quantum Healing: Exploring the Frontiers of Mind/Body Medicine*. New York: Bantam Books. 1989.

Chopra, Deepak, MD. *Ageless Body, Timeless Mind: The Quantum Alternative to Growing Old*. New York: Harmony Books. 1993.

Chopra, Deepak, MD. *Unconditional Life: Mastering the Forces That Shape Personal Reality*. New York: Bantam Books. 1991.

Weil, Andrew, MD. *Spontaneous Healing: How to Discover and Enhance Your Body's Natural Ability to Maintain and Heal Itself*. New York: Alfred A. Knopf. 1995.

Weil, Andrew MD. *Health and Healing*. Boston: Houghton Mifflin Co. 1988.

Wilber, Ken. *Grace and Grit: Spirituality and Healing in the Life and Death of Treya Killam Wilber*. Boston: Shambhala. 1993.

Wilber, Ken. *The Spectrum of Consciousness*. Wheaton, IL: Theosophical Publishing House. 1982.

Wilber, Ken. *No Boundary: Eastern and Western Approaches to Personal Growth*. Boston: Shambhala. 1979.

Wilber, Ken. *The Marriage of Sense and Soul. Integrating Science and Religion*. New York: Broadway Books. 1988.

Hanh, Thich Nhat. *The Heart of the Buddha's Teaching: Transforming Suffering into Peace, Joy, and Liberation*. New York: Broadway Books. 1999.

Chodron, Pema. *When Things Fall Apart: Heart Advice for Difficult Times*. Boston: Shambhala. 1997.

Ram Dass. *Be Here Now*. New York: Crown Publishers. 1971

Ram Dass (compiler). *Miracle of Love. Stories About Neem Karoli Baba*. Santa Fe, NM: Hanuman Foundation. 1995.

Barasch, Marc Ian. *The Healing Path. A Soul Approach to Illness*. New York: Penguin Books. 1993.

Moore, Thomas. *Care of the Soul: A Guide for Cultivating Depth and Sacredness in Everyday Life*. New York: HarperCollins. 1992.

Naparstek, Belleruth. *Your Sixth Sense: Activating Your Psychic Potential*. New York: HarperSanFrancisco/HarperCollins Publishers, Inc. 1997.

Harpham, Wendy Schlessel, MD. *After Cancer: A Guide to Your New Life*. New York: W. W. Norton and Co. 1994.

Havorson-Boyd, Glenna, and Hunter, Lisa K. *Dancing in Limbo: Making Sense of Life After Cancer*. San Francisco: Jossey-Bass, Inc. 1995.

Radner, Gilda. *It's Always Something*. New York: Avon. 1995.

Canfield, Jack, and Hansen, Mark Victor. *Chicken Soup for the Soul: 101 Stories to Open the Heart and Rekindle the Spirit.* Deerfield Beach, FL: Health Communications, Inc. 1996.

Canfield, Jack; Hansen, Mark Victor; Aubery, Patty; and Mitchell, Nancy, RN. *Chicken Soup for the Surviving Soul: 101 Stories of Courage and Inspiration from Those Who Have Survived Cancer.* Deerfield Beach, FL: Health Communications, Inc. 1996.

Anderson, Gregg. *Healing Wisdom: Wit, Insight and Inspiration for Anyone Facing Illness.* New York: Penguin Books. 1994.

Anderson, Gregg. *The 22 {Non-Negotiable} Laws of Wellness: Feel, Think, and Live Better Than You Ever Thought Possible.* New York: HarperCollins. 1995.

Carlson, Richard, PhD. *Don't Sweat the Small Stuff…and It's All Small Stuff: Simple Ways to Stop the Little Things from Taking over Your Life.* New York: Hyperion. 1997.

Clifford, Christine. *Not Now…I'm Having a No Hair Day: Humor & Healing for People with Cancer.* Duluth, MN: Pfeifer-Hamilton Publishers. 1996.

Becton, Randy. *Everyday Strength: A Cancer Patient's Guide to Spiritual Survival.* Grand Rapids, MI: Baker Books. 1989.

Hayward, Susan. *A Guide for the Advanced Soul: A Book of Insight.* Boston: Little Brown and Company. 1995.

Brennan, Barbara Ann. *Light Emerging: The Journey of Personal Healing.* New York: Bantam Books. 1993.

Topf, Linda Noble, MA. *You Are Not Your Illness: Seven Principles for Meeting the Challenge.* New York: Simon & Schuster. 1995.

A Course in Miracles. Tiburon, CA: Foundation for Inner Peace. 1975.

Williamson, Marianne. *A Return to Love: Reflections on the Principles of a Course in Miracles.* New York: HarperCollins. 1992.

Vaughan, Frances, PhD, and Walsh, Roger, MD, PhD. *A Gift of Peace: Selections from a Course in Miracles.* Los Angeles: Jeremy P. Tarcher. 1986.

Vaughn, Frances, PhD. *Shadows of the Sacred: Seeing Through Spiritual Illusions.* Wheaton, IL: Quest Books. 1995.

Walsh, Roger, MD, PhD, and Vaughan, Frances, PhD (editors). *Paths Beyond Ego: The Transpersonal Vision.* New York: G.P. Putnam's Sons. 1993.

Levine, Stephen and Ondrea. *Embracing the Beloved: Relationship as a Path of Awakening.* New York: Doubleday. 1995.

Welwood, John, PhD. *Love and Awakening: Discovering the Sacred Path of Intimate Relationship.* New York: HarperCollins. 1996.

Welwood, John, PhD. *Journey of the Heart: Intimate Relationship and the Path of Love.* New York: HarperCollins. 1990.

Gawain, Shakti, with King, Laurel. *Living in the Light: A Guide to Personal and Planetary Transformation.* San Rafael, CA: New World Library. 1986.

The Institute of Noetic Sciences, with William Poole. *The Heart of Healing.* Atlanta: Turner Publishing, Inc. 1993.

Carlson, Richard and Shield, Benjamin. *Handbook for the Soul.* Boston: Little, Brown & Company. 1995.

B. TAPES

The following cassette tapes provide wonderful guidance for deep relaxation, visualization, guided imagery, and self-healing for patients and families.

1. *Health Journeys: For People with Cancer.* Belleruth Naparstek. Time Warner AudioBooks. Los Angeles, CA. 1993.
2. *Health Journeys: For People Undergoing Chemotherapy.* Belleruth Naparstek. Time Warner AudioBooks. Los Angeles, CA. 1993.
3. *Health Journeys: For People Experiencing Stress.* Belleruth Naparstek. Time Warner AudioBooks. Los Angeles, CA. 1995.
4. *Health Journeys: For People with Depression.* Belleruth Naparstek. Time Warner AudioBooks. Los Angeles, CA. 1993.
5. *Health Journeys: For People Experiencing Grief.* Belleruth Naparstek. Time Warner AudioBooks. Los Angeles, CA. 1993.
6. *Health Journeys: For People Managing Pain.* Belleruth Naparstek. Time Warner AudioBooks. Los Angeles, CA. 1995.
7. *Creative Visualization: Meditations from the Book.* Shakti Gawain. New World Library. San Rafael, CA. 1995.
8. *Self-Healing: Creating Your Health, Loving Yourself.* Louise L. Hay. Hay House Audio. Carlsbad, CA. 1983.
9. *Contacting Your Inner Healer: A Guided Imagery Relaxation Tape with Action Plan.* Neil F. Neimark, MD. R.E.P. Technologies. 1998.
10. *Effective Meditations for Stress Relief.* Contemporary Meditation Series. Effective Learning Systems. Port Richmond, CA. 1995.
11. *The Miracle of Mindfulness: A Manual on Meditation.* Abridged Audio Cassettes: Thich Nhat Hanh. Harper Audio. Carlsbad, CA. 1995.
12. *Healing Journey.* Marci Archambeault. The Quest. Leominster, MA. 1996.
13. *Peaceful Body, Quiet Mind: A Healing Program of Curative Images, Positive Affirmations, and Serene Music/Cassette.* Harriett Sanders. New Harbinger Publishers. Oakland, CA. 1995.
14. *Meditation for Beginners.* Jack Kornfield. Sounds True. Louisville, CO. 1998.

15. *The Inner Art of Meditation.* Jack Kornfield. Sounds True. Louisville, CO. 1997.
16. *How to Meditate.* Lawrence LeShan. Audio Forum. Gilford, CT. 1987.
17. *Deep Relaxation/Audio Cassette.* Robert Griswold. Effective Learning Systems. Port Richmond, CA. 1992.
18. *Effective Meditations for Health and Healing.* Meditation Contemporary. Effective Learning Systems. Bonita Springs, FL. 1995.

C. CDs

The following CDs contain warm, soothing music to facilitate rest, relaxation, meditation, healing, and the experience of joy and inner peace.

1. *Cristofori's Dream.* David Lanz. Essex Music. Milwaukee, WI. 1988.
2. *The Silent Path.* Robert Haig Coxon. RHC Productions, Inc. Quebec, Canada. 1995.
3. *In the Enchanted Garden.* Kevin Kern. Real Music. Sausalito, CA. 1996.
4. *Following the Circle.* Dik Darnell. Variena Music. Littleton, CO. 1988.
5. *O'cean: Flute Music with Humpback Whale Sounds.* Larkin. Narada Promotions, Inc. Milwaukee, WI. 1985.
6. *Celtic Spirit: Narada Collection Series.* Milwaukee, WI: Celtic Legacy/Narada Media. 1996.
7. *Chant: The Benedictine Monks of Santo Domingo de Silos.* Hispavox. Madrid, Spain. 1973.
8. *The Magic of Healing Music, Vata: Relaxing.* Created for Deepak Chopra. Bruce BecVar and Brian BecVar. Gus Swigert Management. 1995.
9. *The Magic of Healing Music, Pitta: Calming.* Created for Deepak Chopra. Bruce BecVar and Brian BecVar. Gus Swigert Management. 1995.
10. *The Magic of Healing Music, Kapha: Invigorating.* Created for Deepak Chopra. Bruce BecVar and Brian BecVar. Gus Swigert Management. 1995.
11. *Pasayadan and Mahalakshmi Stotram: As Sung in Siddha Yoga Meditation Ashrams.* SYDA Foundation. South Fallsburg, NY. 1994.
12. *Chants of India.* Produced by George Harrison. Ravi Shankar. Angel Records. New York, NY. 1997.

APPENDIX 2: CANCER SUPPORT ORGANIZATIONS

American Brain Tumor Association
2720 River Road
Des Plaines, IL 60018
(847) 827-9910
(800) 886-ABTA (800-886-2282)

American Cancer Society
   National Headquarters
1599 Clifton Road, N.E.
Atlanta, GA 30329
(800) ACS-2345

American Foundation for
   Urological Disease
300 West Pratt St., Suite 401
Baltimore, MD 21201
(410) 727-2908
(800) 828-7866

American Pain Society
4700 West Lake Avenue
Glenview, IL 60025
(847) 375-4715

American Society of Clinical Oncology
225 Reineckers Lane, Suite 650
Alexandria, VA 22314
(703) 299-0150

Bone Marrow Transplant Family
   Support Network
P.O. Box 845
Avon, CT 06001
(800) 826-9376

Brain Tumor Society
84 Seattle St.
Boston, MA 02134
(617) 783-0340
(800) 770-8287

Caitlin Raymond International
   (Bone Marrow) Registry
University of Massachusetts
   Medical Center
55 Lake Avenue North
Worcester, MA 01655
(508) 756-6444
(800) 7-AMATCH (800-726-2824)

Cancer Care, Inc.
1180 Avenue of the Americas
New York, NY 10036
(212) 302-2400
(800) 813-4673

Cancer Control Society
2043 North Verendo Street
Los Angeles, CA 90027
(800) 227-2345

Cancer Information Service
National Cancer Institute
Building 31, Room 10A16
9000 Rockville Pike
Bethesda, MD 20892
(800) 4-CANCER (800-422-6237)

Cancervive
6500 Wilshire Blvd., Suite 500
Los Angeles, CA 90048
(310) 203-9232

Candlelighters Childhood Cancer
  Foundation
7910 Woodmont Avenue, Suite 460
Bethesda, MD 20814
(301) 657-8401
(800) 366-2223

CANHELP
3111 Paradise Bay Road
Port Ludlow, WA 98365
(360) 437-2291

CaPCURE
1250 Fourth St., Suite 360
Santa Monica, CA 90401
(310) 458-2873
(800) 757-2873

Center for Attitudinal Healing
33 Buchanan Drive
Sausalito, CA 94965
(415) 331-6161

Children's Hospice International
2202 Mt. Vernon Avenue, Suite 3C
Alexandria, VA 22301
(703) 684-0330
(800) 242-4453

Commonweal
Cancer Help Program
P.O. Box 316
Bolinas, CA 94924
(415) 868-0970

Corporate Angel Network
Westchester County Airport
Building One
White Plains, NY 10604
(914) 328-1313

Cure for Lymphoma Foundation
215 Lexington Avenue
New York, NY 10016
(212) 213-9595

Exceptional Cancer Patients
522 Jackson Park Drive
Meadeville, PA 16335
(814) 337-8192

Gilda Radner Familial Ovarian
  Cancer Registry
Roswell Park Cancer Institute
Elm and Carlton Streets
Buffalo, NY 14263
(800) 682-7426

Healing Choices
144 St. John's Place
Brooklyn, NY 11217
(718) 636-1679

Hospice Education Institute
190 Westbrook Road
Essex, CT 06426
(203) 767-1620
(800) 331-1620

International Association for
    Enterostomal Therapy
505-A Tustin Avenue, Suite 282
Santa Ana, CA 92705
(714) 972-1725

International Association of
    Laryngectomies
1599 Clifton Road N.E.
Atlanta, GA 30329
(404) 329-7650

International Myeloma Foundation
2120 Stanley Hills Drive
Los Angeles, CA 90046
(213) 654-3023
(800) 452-CURE (800-452-2873)

Leukemia Society of America
600 Third Avenue
New York, NY 10016
(212) 573-8484
(800) 955-4572

Lymphoma Foundation of America
PO Box 15335
Chevy Chase, MD 20825
(202) 223-6181

Make-a-Wish Foundation of America
100 West Clarendon, Suite 2200
Phoenix, AZ 85013
(602) 279-9474
(800) 722-WISH (800-722-9474)

Melanoma Center
UCSF/Mt. Zion Medical Center
2356 Sutter Street, 5th Floor
San Francisco, CA 94115
(415) 885-7546

National Alliance of Breast
    Cancer Organizations
9 East 37th Street, 10th Floor
New York, NY 10016
(212) 719-0154
(800) 719-9154

National Breast Cancer Coalition
1707 L. Street, N.W., Suite 1060
Washington, DC 20036
(202) 296-7477
(800) 622-2838

National Cancer Institute
Building 31, Room 10A19
9000 Rockville Pike
Bethesda, MD 20892
(800) 4-CANCER (800-422-6237)

National Center for Complementary
    and Alternative Medicine
NCCAM Clearinghouse
PO Box 8218
Silver Spring, MD 20907
(888) 644-6226

National Coalition for Cancer
    Survivorship
101 Wayne Avenue, 5th Floor
Silver Spring, MD 20910
(310) 650-8868

National Family Caregivers
  Association
10400 Connecticut Ave., Suite 500
Kensington, MD 20895
(301) 942-6430
(800) 896-3650

National Hospice Organization
1901 N. Moore Street, Suite 901
Arlington, VA 22209
(703) 243-5900
(800) 658-8898

National Leukemia Research
  Association
585 Stewart Avenue, Suite 536
Garden City, NY 11530
(516) 222-1944

National Lymphedema Network
2211 Post Street, Suite 404
San Francisco, CA 94115
(415) 921-1306
(800) 541-3259

National Ovarian Cancer Coalition
500 Spanish River Blvd., Suite 14
Boca Raton, FL 33431
(561) 393-0005
(888) 683-7426

National Patient Air
  Transport Hotline
PO Box 2940
Manassas, VA 20108
(703) 361-1191
(800) 296-1217

Patient Advocate Foundation
780 Pilot House Dr., Suite 100-C
Newport News, VA 23606
(757) 873-6668
(800) 532-5274

Patient Advocates for Advanced
  Cancer Treatments
1143 Parmelee N.W.
Grand Rapids, MI 49504
(616) 453-1477

People Against Cancer
PO Box 10
604 East Street
Otho, IA 50569
(515) 972-4444

Planetree Health Resource Center
2040 Webster Street
San Francisco, CA 94115
(415) 923-3680

Ronald McDonald House Charities
One Kroc Drive
Oak Brook, IL 60523
(630) 623-7048

Smith Farm Center for the
  Healing Arts
1229 Fifteenth St. NW
Washington, DC 20005
(202) 483-8601

Skin Cancer Foundation
245 Fifth Avenue, Suite 1403
New York, NY 10016
(212) 725-5176

Susan G. Komen Breast Cancer
  Foundation
5005 LBJ Freeway, Suite 370
Dallas, TX 75244
(972) 385-5000
(972) 855-1600
(800) IM-AWARE (800-462-9273)

United Ostomy Association
19772 MacArthur Blvd., Suite 200
Irvine, CA 92612
(714) 660-8624
(800) 826-0826

US TOO International
930 North York Road, Suite 50
Hinsdale, IL 60521
(630) 323-1002
(800) 808-7866

Visiting Nurse Association of America
3801 E. Florida Avenue, #900
Denver, CA 80210
(888) 866-8773

Wellness Community National
  Headquarters
2716 Ocean Park Boulevard,
  Suite 1040
Santa Monica, CA 90405
(310) 314-2555

Y-ME National Breast Cancer
  Organization
212 West Van Buren Street, 5th Floor
Chicago, IL 60607
(312) 986-8338
(800) 221-2141

APPENDIX 3: CANCER INFORMATION RESOURCES ON THE INTERNET

The World Wide Web is an extraordinary source of information about cancer, cancer treatment, health, and wellness for patients, family members, caregivers, and friends. Here is a list of some of the best Web sites that may be of assistance to you.

GENERAL INFORMATION SITES

The National Cancer Institute
   (http://www.cancer.gov)
OncoLink: The University of Pennsylvania Cancer Center Resource
   (http://www.oncolink.com)
CANSearch: National Coalition for Cancer Survivorship
   (http://www.cansearch.org)
InterNet Resources for Cancer
   (http://www.ncl.ac.uk/child-health/guides/clinks1.htm)
CancerWEB
   (http://www.graylab.ac.uk/cancerweb)
CancerDirectory
   (http://www.cancerdirectory.com)
Association of Cancer Online Resources
   (http://www.acor.org)
Ask NOAH About: Cancer
   (http://www.noah.cuny.edu/cancer/cancer.html)
CancerGuide: Steve Dunn's Cancer Information Page
   (http://www.cancerguide.org)

American Society of Clinical Oncology
    (http://www.asco.org)
American Cancer Society
    (http://www.cancer.org)
Cancer Care, Inc.
    (http://www.cancercare.org)
Association of Community Cancer Centers
    (http://www.assoc-cancer-ctrs.org)
Cancer News
    (http://www.cancernews.com)
Medicine OnLine
    (http://www.meds.com)
HealthWorld Online
    (http://www.healthy.net)
HealthGate
    (http://www.healthgate.com)
The Health Network
    (http://www.ahn.com)
Yahoo!-Health
    (http://health.yahoo.com)

SITES FOR SPECIFIC TYPES OF CANCER

National Alliance of Breast Cancer Organizations (NABCO)
    (http://www.nabco.org)
National Action Plan on Breast Cancer
    (http://www.napbc.org)
National Breast Cancer Coalition
    (http://www.natlbcc.org)
Susan G. Komen Breast Cancer Foundation
    (http://www.komen.org)
Y-ME National Breast Cancer Oganization
    (http://www.yme.org)
Prostate Cancer Research Institute
    (http://www.prostate-cancer.org)
The National Prostate Cancer Coalition
    (http://www.4npcc.org)
US TOO International, Inc.
    (http://www.ustoo.com)
Cancer Care's Section on Colon Cancer
    (http://www.cancercare.org/campaigns/colon1.htm)

CDC's Section on Colorectal Cancer
   (http://www.cdc.gov/cancer/colorctl/colorect.htm)
Lung Cancer Awareness Campaign
   (http://www.lungcancer.org)
Cancer Care's Section on Lung Cancer
   (http://www.cancercare.org/campaigns/lungcancer1.htm)
National Ovarian Cancer Coalition
   (http://www.ovarian.org)
Gilda Radner Familial Ovarian Cancer Registry
   (http://rpci.med.buffalo.edu/clinic/gynonc/grwp.html)
Pancreas Cancer Home Page
   (http://www.path.jhu.edu/pancreas)
American Brain Tumor Association
   (http://www.abta.org)
Lymphoma Research Foundation of America, Inc.
   (http://www.lymphoma.org)
Leukemia Society of America
   (http://www.leukemia.org)
The International Myeloma Foundation
   (http://www.myeloma.org)
The Myelodysplastic Syndromes (MDS) Foundation
   (http://www.mds-foundation.org)
National Cervical Cancer Coalition
   (http://www.nccc-online.org)
National Bone Marrow Transplant Link
   (http://www.comnet.org/nbmtlink)

COMPLEMENTARY AND ALTERNATIVE MEDICINE

National Center for Complementary and Alternative Medicine
   (http://nccam.nih.gov)
Center for Alternative Medicine Research in Cancer
   (http://www.sph.uth.tmc.edu/utcam)
Alternative Health News Online
   (http://www.altmedicine.com)
WellnessWeb Alternative/Complementary Medicine
   (http://www.wellweb.com/alternativecomplementary_medicine.htm)
Alternative Medicine
   (http://www.alternativemedicine.com)
Commonweal
   (http://www.commonweal.org)

APPENDIX 4: NCI-DESIGNATED COMPREHENSIVE CANCER CENTERS

The following have been designated as "comprehensive cancer centers" by the National Cancer Institute.

ALABAMA

University of Alabama at Birmingham
Comprehensive Cancer Center
1824 Sixth Avenue South
Birmingham, AL 35294
(205) 975-8222

ARIZONA

University of Arizona Cancer Center
1501 North Campbell Avenue
Tucson, AZ 85724
(520) 626-6044

CALIFORNIA

City of Hope National Medical Center
   and Beckman Research Institute
1500 East Duarte Road
Duarte, CA 91010
(626) 359-8111

Jonsson Comprehensive Cancer Center
University of California at Los Angeles
10833 Le Conte Avenue
Los Angeles, CA 90095
(310) 825-2631

Norris Comprehensive Cancer Center
University of Southern California
1441 Eastlake Avenue
Los Angeles, CA 90033
(323) 865-3000

Chao Family Comprehensive
   Cancer Center
University of California at Irvine
101 The City Drive
Orange, CA 92868
(714) 456-8000

COLORADO

University of Colorado Cancer Center
4200 East 9th Avenue, Box B188
Denver, CO 80262
(303) 315-3007

CONNECTICUT

Yale University School of Medicine
Comprehensive Cancer Center
333 Cedar Street
New Haven, CT 06520
(203) 785-4095

DISTRICT OF COLUMBIA

Lombardi Cancer Research Center
Georgetown University Medical
    Center
3800 Reservoir Road N.W.
Washington, DC 20007
(202) 687-2110

FLORIDA

H. Lee Moffitt Cancer Center
    and Research Institute
12902 Magnolia Drive
Tampa, FL 33612
(813) 972-4673

ILLINOIS

University of Chicago Cancer
    Research Center
5841 South Maryland Avenue,
    MC 1140
Chicago, IL 60637
(773) 702-9200

Robert H. Lurie Cancer Center
Northwestern University
303 East Chicago Avenue
Chicago, IL 60611
(312) 908-5250

MARYLAND

Johns Hopkins Oncology Center
600 North Wolfe Street
Baltimore, MD 21287
(410) 955-5000

MASSACHUSETTS

Dana-Farber Cancer Institute
44 Binney Street
Boston, MA 02115
(617) 632-3000

MICHIGAN

Comprehensive Cancer Center
University of Michigan
1500 East Medical Center Drive
Ann Arbor, MI 48109
(734) 936-2516

Barbara Ann Karmanos
    Cancer Institute
Wayne State University
110 East Warren
Detroit, MI 48201
(313) 993-7777

MINNESOTA

University of Minnesota
    Cancer Center
Box 806, 420 Delaware Street, S.E.
Minneapolis, MN 55455
(612) 624-8484

Mayo Clinic Cancer Center
200 First Street, S.W.
Rochester, MN 55905
(507) 284-9589

NEW HAMPSHIRE

Norris Cotton Cancer Center
Dartmouth-Hitchcock Medical Center
One Medical Center Drive
Lebanon, NH 03756
(603) 650-5000

NEW YORK

Comprehensive Cancer Center
Albert Einstein College of Medicine
1300 Morris Park Avenue
Bronx, NY 10461
(718) 430-2302

Roswell Park Cancer Institute
Elm and Carlton Streets
Buffalo, NY 14263
(716) 845-2300

Kaplan Cancer Center
New York University Medical Center
550 First Avenue
New York, NY 10016
(212) 263-6485

Memorial Sloan-Kettering Cancer
  Center
1275 York Avenue
New York, NY 10021
(212) 639-2000

Herbert Irving Comprehensive
  Cancer Center
College of Physicians & Surgeons
Columbia University
177 Fort Washington Avenue
New York, NY 10032
(212) 305-8602

NORTH CAROLINA

UNC Lineberger Comprehensive
  Cancer Center
University of North Carolina School of
  Medicine
102 West Drive
Chapel Hill, NC 27599-7295
(919) 966-3036

Duke Comprehensive Cancer Center
Duke University Medical Center
Box 3843
Durham, NC 27710
(919) 684-3377

Comprehensive Cancer Center
Wake Forest University Baptist
  Medical Center
Medical Center Boulevard
Winston-Salem, NC 27157
(336) 716-2075

OHIO

Ireland Cancer Center
Case Western Reserve University and
  University Hospitals of Cleveland
11100 Euclid Avenue
Cleveland, OH 44106
(216) 844-5432

Comprehensive Cancer Center
Arthur G. James Cancer Hospital
Ohio State University
300 West 10th Avenue
Columbus, OH 43210
(614) 293-5485

PENNSYLVANIA

University of Pennsylvania Cancer
  Center
3400 Spruce Street
Philadelphia, PA 19104
(215) 662-7979

Fox Chase Cancer Center
7701 Burholme Avenue
Philadelphia, PA 19111
(215) 728-6900

University of Pittsburgh
  Cancer Institute
3471 Fifth Avenue, Suite 201
Pittsburgh, PA 15213
(412) 692-4670

TEXAS

M.D. Anderson Cancer Center
University of Texas
1515 Holcombe Boulevard
Houston, TX 77030
(713) 792-2121

San Antonio Cancer Institute
8122 Datapoint Drive, Suite 600
San Antonio, TX 78229
(210) 616-5590

VERMONT

Vermont Cancer Center
University of Vermont
Medical Alumni Building, 2nd Floor
Burlington, VT 05405
(802) 656-4414

WASHINGTON

Fred Hutchinson Cancer Research
  Center
1100 Fairview Avenue, North
Seattle, WA 98104
(206) 667-4324

WISCONSIN

Comprehensive Cancer Center
University of Wisconsin
600 Highland Avenue
Madison, WI 53792
(608) 262-5223

INDEX

ABOUT THE AUTHOR

JEREMY R. GEFFEN, M.D., F.A.C.P., is the founder and director of the Geffen Cancer Center and Research Institute in Vero Beach, Florida (www.geffencenter.com). He is a board-certified medical oncologist and a Fellow of the American College of Physicians. Dr. Geffen is a summa cum laude graduate of Columbia University and received his M.D. degree with honors from New York University School of Medicine. He completed residency training in internal medicine at the University of California at San Diego Medical Center and fellowship training in hematology and oncology at the University of California at San Francisco Medical Center. Dr. Geffen has also traveled extensively and has more than twenty-five years of experience exploring the great spiritual and healing traditions of the East, including Ayurveda, Tibetan Medicine, yoga, meditation, and other approaches to self-awareness. Along with his work at the center, he lectures widely on the mind/body aspects of cancer and the emerging new paradigm of medicine.